Outcome Measurement and Management: First Steps for the Practicing Clinician

Outcome Measurement and Management:

First Steps for the Practicing Clinician

Sandra L. Kaplan, PT, PhD
Associate Professor and Assistant Director,
Doctoral Programs in Physical Therapy
Member Stuart D. Cook MD Master Educators Guild
University of Medicine and Dentistry of New Jersey
Newark, New Jersey

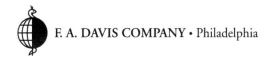
F. A. DAVIS COMPANY • Philadelphia

F. A. Davis Company
1915 Arch Street
Philadelphia, PA 19103
www.fadavis.com

Printed in the United States of America

Last digit indicates print number: 10 9 8 7 6 5 4 3 2 1

Acquisitions Editor: Margaret Biblis
Developmental Editor: Jennifer Pine
Manager of Art & Design: Carolyn O'Brien

As new scientific information becomes available through basic and clinical research, recommended treatments and drug therapies undergo changes. The authors and publisher have done everything possible to make this book accurate, up to date, and in accord with accepted standards at the time of publication. The authors, editors, and publisher are not responsible for errors or omissions or for consequences from application of the book, and make no warranty, expressed or implied, in regard to the contents of the book. Any practice described in this book should be applied by the reader in accordance with professional standards of care used in regard to the unique circumstances that may apply in each situation. The reader is advised always to check product information (package inserts) for changes and new information regarding dose and contraindications before administering any drug. Caution is especially urged when using new or infrequently ordered drugs.

Library of Congress Cataloging-in-Publication Data

Kaplan, Sandra L.
    Outcome measurement and management: first steps for the praticing clinician/
  Sandra L. Kaplan.
      p. ; cm.
    ISBN-13: 978-0-8036-0310-3 (alk. paper)
    ISBN-10: 0-8036-0310-X (alk. paper)
    1. Medical rehabilitation. 2. Outcome assessment (Medical care)
I. Title.
  [DNLM: 1. Rehabilitation. 2. Treatment Outcome. 3. Data Collection
—methods. 4. Data Interpretation, Statistical. 5. Patient Care Planning
—organization & administration. 6.Physician Practice Patterns.
WB 320 K17f 2007]
RM930.K37 2007
362.1—dc22   2006013289

To Steve,
for your constant support,
and to our two most important outcomes,
Kayla and Eric,
who challenge my assumptions on a daily basis.

Preface

This book has two main goals:

GOAL 1: TO INTRODUCE READERS TO THE TERMINOLOGY AND PROCESSES OF OUTCOME MEASUREMENT

This first goal may seem straightforward enough. At the time I began this project (mid-1990s), there were very few books that addressed outcome measurement in rehabilitation. In fact, most of the literature available was, and continues to be, in the domains of medicine, nursing, and quality assurance. Pulling definitions together, finding threads to tie processes together, and finding links to the educational and experiential backgrounds of physical therapists have and continue to be an iterative process of new discovery, reorganization, and refinement.

This book does not purport to be an exhaustive review of the literature. Rather, it uses literature to credit ideas, provide examples, and demonstrate the range of strategies available to address outcome measurement processes. I have tried to pick examples from the literature that illustrate ideas and that also represent the wide variety of practice venues of physical therapists.

Many of the ideas and suggestions provided in this book are my own, having evolved from conducting outcome studies and teaching courses on outcome measurement. I have had the privilege of teaching these courses to professional and post-professional physical therapy students. Many explanations that have been included are there because students needed "dots" to be explained or "dots" to be connected. I am grateful to the many students who have asked questions and shared their confusions, as they have helped to ground the application of information in practical terms.

I have also learned that while the academic community is immersed in such frameworks and terminology as *disablement models*, *evidence-based practice*, and *measurable outcomes,* there are many practicing clinicians who have not applied or observed these frameworks or terms in their daily clinical practice. Recognizing the categories of a disablement model appears to be a different skill than categorizing examination measures according to that model or using the model to create hypotheses about patient care. Consequently, I have included chapters about service delivery models, disablement models, and statistics. Academic programs teach this content in greater depth, so current students and recent graduates may not need these chapters. They have been included to help those practicing clinicians who have not had the same academic exposure and to enable clinicians from other professions to use that information.

GOAL 2: TO PROVIDE CLINICIANS WITH STRATEGIES FOR USING THEIR OWN DOCUMENTATION TO EVALUATE THEIR PRACTICE PATTERNS OR EFFECTIVENESS RETROSPECTIVELY

This second goal was the harder of the two to address, and I am hopeful that Part 2 of this book successfully delivers on the goal. Outcome measurement/management is the convergence of two traditional curricular tracks found in most professional PT programs: the scientific inquiry/research track and the administration/health policy track. In traditional scientific inquiry/research tracks, students learn about research designs, statistics, and critical literature review processes. They apply these skills to clinical questions, using the steps of evidence-based practice or the traditional thesis process. Administration courses address federal and state regulations, service delivery models, and the nuts and bolts of running a department or private practice. Outcome measurement is the process of applying scientific inquiry skills to service delivery challenges in the hopes of improving patient outcomes. This convergence of the two curricular tracks is not often explicit in professional curricula; however, the realities of the current practice environment are requiring clinicians to access data for clinical decision-making, performance benchmarking, and developing or evaluating clinical pathways and guidelines.

This book introduces the beginning of the process—a means for objectively evaluating a clinician's own practice and of validating assumptions about how clinicians document what is done with patients and at what levels of effectiveness. The purpose of the exercises is to have clinicians use their own patient pool as a laboratory for self-analysis. When a clinician is sensitized to the challenges of objective, repeated, and complete documentation, the clinician will be better prepared to look at the quality of available data and what they can say about patient care.

NOTE: THIS BOOK WILL NOT TEACH READERS ABOUT DESIGNING OR CONDUCTING PROSPECTIVE STUDIES.

This book is not designed to teach the reader how to conduct prospective research with patient populations. Designing studies before collecting data requires many more layers of preparation, knowledge, and process than do retrospective chart reviews for informing clinical decision making. Clinicians who have been "bitten by the research bug" are highly encouraged to pursue advanced training through collaboration with clinical researchers or academic programs.

Reviewers

Diana M. Bailey, EdD, OTR, FAOTA
Associate Professor
Occupational Therapy Program
Tufts University
Medford, Massachusetts

Suzanne R. Brown, PT, MPH
Chair and Associate Professor
Physical Therapy Department
Arizona School of Health Sciences
Mesa, Arizona

Sandra L. Cassidy, PT, PhD, FAACVPR
Professor and Director
Physical Therapy Department
St. Ambrose University
Davenport, Iowa

D. Scott Davis, PT, MS, OCS
Assistant Professor
Physical Therapy Department
West Virginia University
Morgantown, West Virginia

Kristen Geissler, PT, MS
Rehabilitation Sciences Department
University of Maryland–Baltimore
Baltimore, Maryland

Steven Z. George, PT, PhD, MS
Assistant Professor
Physical Therapy Department
University of Florida
Gainesville, Florida

John H. Hollman, PT, PhD
Assistant Professor
Physical Therapy Program
Mayo School of Health Sciences
Rochester, Minnesota

Pamela K. Levangie, PT, DSC
Associate Professor
Physical Therapy Department
Sacred Heart University
Fairfield, Connecticut

Sandy Marden-Lokken, PT, MA
Assistant Professor
Physical Therapy Department
The College of St. Scholastica
Duluth, Minnesota

Roger M. Nelson, PT, PhD, FAPTA
Professor
Physical Therapy Department
Lebanon Valley College
Annville, Pennsylvania

Cynthia C. Norkin, PT, EdD
(Retired)
Former Director and Associate
    Professor
Physical Therapy Department
Ohio University
Athens, Ohio

Jan F. Perry, PT, EdD
(Retired)
Former Chairman and Professor
Physical Therapy Department
Medical College of Georgia
Augusta, Georgia

Michael J. Rennick, PT, MPH
Assistant Professor
Physical Therapy Education
University of Nebraska Medical
    Center
Omaha, Nebraska

Linda J. Resnik, PT, PhD, OCS
Assistant Professor
Community Health Department
Brown University
Providence, Rhode Island

Thomas J. Schmitz, PT, PhD
Assistant Professor
Division of Physical Therapy
Long Island University
Brooklyn, New York

Andrew J. Strubhar, PT, PhD
Associate Professor
Physical Therapy and Health
  Sciences Department
Bradley University
Peoria, Illinois

Frank B. Underwood, PT, PhD, ECS
Professor
Physical Therapy Department
University of Evansville
Evansville, Indiana

Denise Wise, PT, PhD
Chair and Associate Professor
Physical Therapy Department
The College of St. Scholastica
Duluth, Minnesota

Acknowledgments

I thank the many people who have supported my efforts on this project since the seed was first planted. Thank you, Roger Nelson, for recruiting me onto an APTA task force to study outcomes in physical therapy. That started me on this jigsaw puzzle, and I am only now beginning to figure out where the edges are! Thank you to the FA Davis family: Jean-Francois Vilain, who first reached out to me about the idea for a book, and to Margaret Biblis and Jennifer Pine, who caught the project midair and helped to land it in its current form. Thank you to my friend and administrative mentor, Alma Merians, who found creative ways to support my phases of academic myopia needed to finish this book. Thank you to my faculty peers: our curricular discussions and the opportunities to teach my courses on Outcome Measurement and Management have informed the book's scope and content. Thank you to the many students who have taken my courses, read drafts of these chapters, and provided valuable feedback. Thank you, George Gabriel, for agreeing to have your class assignment be used as an example.

Brief Contents

Contents

PART 3

Integrating Outcome Measurement and Clinical Practice   181

Preface to Part 3

Chapter 13 • Considerations for Conducting Outcome Studies

Chapter 14 • Mixing Outcome Measurement With Practice Management

APPENDICES

## PART 1

DEFINING OUTCOMES IN CLINICAL PRACTICE

An Introduction to Outcome Measurement and Management

KEY TERMS

Outcome research

Data collector

Documentation

Cohort data

Retrospective chart review

CHAPTER OUTCOMES

➤ Appreciate the need to document objective data in clinical practice systematically.

➤ Contrast the steps of patient care management with outcome research processes.

➤ Describe the challenges of using clinical documentation as a source for retrospective case studies and cohort data.

"Am I an effective clinician?"
"How many of my patients achieve their goals?"
"Are my patients satisfied with their gains?"
"Can my treatments be more efficient or effective?"

These are the questions that drive a reflective practitioner. There are many definitions of "effective," and there are many strategies for reviewing a clinician's individual decision-making processes. This textbook will guide the physical therapist (PT) through one method of evaluating clinical practice by using daily documentation as a source for retrospective data. By **looking backward**, a clinician will be able to compare intuitive perceptions of process or effectiveness with objective measures of service delivery.

Every clinician can learn to translate routine patient documentation into data sets in order to measure personal service outcomes. Health service delivery has entered the era of evidence-based practice. Patients, peers, and regulatory agencies are holding health-care providers to a higher level of accountability than ever before. They want measurable evidence that an intervention is yielding positive results for the least amount of money. Consumers and payers want their money's worth, and satisfaction is linked to the achievement of expected results (Keith, 1998; Kramer, 1997; McKinley, et al., 2002). Although the literature supporting physical therapy interventions and outcomes is growing steadily, there is still a dearth of rigorous clinical trials and clinically applicable outcomes that provide clinicians with the published support for many intervention strategies (Delitto, 2005; Duckworth, 1999; Jette, 2005). So, on the one hand, patients, payers, and clinicians want evidence of effectiveness. On the other hand, the literature does not provide the breadth and depth of support for the many problems and approaches that PTs address. What is a clinician to do?

> *A Challenge: Consumers and clinicians want evidence of effectiveness, but there is limited support for many intervention strategies.*

One solution to this dilemma is to view each patient as a case study. The patient becomes a sample of $n=1$ and presents a unique opportunity to test a clinical hypothesis about the best strategy to achieve that patient's goals. Daily documentation on initial patient status and subsequent changes during the course of patient management become the data set. When the measurements on a desired change demonstrate improvement, they support the choice of interventions for this particular patient at this particular time. When the measurements decline or do not change as expected, that evidence supports a change in intervention strategy. Use of patient data for clinical decision making is part of the classical triad of evidence-based practice (Sackett, et al., 2000), but although single case report data are better than pure intuition, they are not the strongest form of evidence.

> *One Solution: each patient is an $n=1$.*

Another solution would be to combine data across several patients who present with the same array of pathology, signs, symptoms, and functional goals. This is only possible if documentation of the measurements taken across patients is consistent. This type of measurement consistency can vary widely unless the documentation forms and collection processes require consistency. When it exists, combining data across patients provides stronger evidence to support clinical decision making than data from a single patient report. Clearly then, the challenge for every clinician is to learn to turn daily documentation into data that can inform clinical decision making; that is the purpose of this book.

> *Another Solution: combine patients so $n=>1$.*

By the end of this chapter, the reader will appreciate the parallels between patient care management and the measurement of outcomes and understand how patient documentation can be used to improve clinical services.

A BRIEF HISTORY OF OUTCOME RESEARCH IN PHYSICAL THERAPY

The need for outcome studies of physical therapy and other rehabilitation services has been, and continues to be, well documented in the literature (Duckworth, 1999; Seelman, 2000). Since 1980, the National Institute on Disability and Rehabilitation Research has funded numerous grants to support the development of outcome measurement tools, studies of interventions and outcomes, educational materials to teach functional outcome measurement, and most recently, the Rehabilitation Research and Training Center for organizing, conducting, and evaluating the application of outcome research to clinical practice (Haley & Jette, 2000; Seelman, 2000). More important, the need for outcome studies is evident in the day-to-day management of patients. When searching for evidence to support patient management strategies, students and clinicians are often surprised to find many studies related to the chosen diagnosis but fewer than they expected on the specific clinical question.

"When will someone tell us what outcome measure to use?"

The initial cries for outcome research in physical therapy began in the mid-1980s and were followed by a flurry of activities. Posters and papers began to appear at conferences and in journals with titles that included the word "outcome." The increased visibility of that term provided a sense of security that the process of outcome measurement was surely going on by some for the sake of many.

PTs often asked how to find the "right" outcome measure, as though there could or should be only one, or they wanted to know how to achieve the best outcome with their patients.

"When is someone going to tell us how to achieve the best outcomes with my patient who has...?"

Clearly there was and continues to be an expectation that someone out there in the professional or scientific community (most probably a PT with a research agenda) would determine the best outcome measures or establish the best practice patterns and share them with the rest of the professional community. And this is happening, as evidenced by the articles, books, and journals that have "outcome" in their title. But in fact, a relatively small percentage of researchers and clinicians are systematically collecting and analyzing outcome data in comparison with the number of clinicians who are practicing. Additionally, the breadth of literature available does not fully represent the variety of the patients who are treated or the variety of environments in which the services are delivered. Often the exclusion criteria used in research designs result in patient samples with similar presentations or severity of symptoms, but these samples are not fully representative of the mix that clinicians see in clinical and community settings. More important, the amount of evidence needed on a daily basis cannot possibly be addressed by the relatively few who are studying the broader clinical issues.

In recent years, the academic spotlight has successively shifted from "outcome research" to "problem-based learning" and most recently to "evidence-based practice," as physical therapy education and professional identity continue to mature. This shifting spotlight may have created the illusion that outcome research is no longer a high priority. In fact, the popularity of evidence-based practice approaches has only served to highlight the fact that just a few of the questions important to PTs have been well studied and that many more have not been addressed as completely or at all. The inability to find answers to specific clinical questions and the need to extrapolate a "best guess" from peripherally related literature often leave the student or clinician a bit frustrated.

THIS BOOK WILL HELP THE INDIVIDUAL CLINICIAN

If a clinician cannot answer any of the following questions, then this book will be a valuable learning tool:

"What are outcomes?"

"Why should I measure them?"

"How do I measure them?"

"What do I do with my results?"

"What are the benefits of studying my outcomes?"

The reader may be a professional or graduate physical therapy student who is learning this material as part of a professional program or as a clinician in the field. Regardless of experience, changes in health-care delivery, reimbursement, and pressure to improve practice through evidence-based decision making, clinical pathways, and benchmarking processes are driving students and clinicians alike to become familiar with outcome measurement processes.

Traditionally, outcome measurement was assumed to be the responsibility of clinical managers or researchers, not the responsibility of staff PTs. That is changing. In the past, staff PTs may have assisted with some of the outcome data collection but often did not design the study or analyze and interpret the data that was collected. Now, consumers and third-party payers are asking individual clinicians for evidence of their intervention effectiveness. They want to know which interventions work the best, which settings get the best results, and which clinicians are most effective. In a sense, consumers want to see a report card on the effectiveness of interventions as well as on the individual clinician or practice setting. This book will be useful to the clinician who does not know where to start an evaluation of clinical effectiveness.

There are many strategies for learning about outcome measurement. Over the past decades, there has been a steady increase in the number of books, websites, journals, and articles dedicated to issues of outcome measurement, most notably in other health-care professions. Workshops, conference presentations, and software that include outcome processes have also become more available. Despite the increased availability of resources, many students and clinicians remain unfamiliar with the basics of outcome measurement. The limitations of time and the desire for an easily digestible overview prevent many from reading individual articles or outcome studies or attending workshops.

This book is an integration of many resources designed to introduce physical therapy students and clinicians to the philosophy and language of outcome measurement. It introduces the basic steps for identifying issues of clinical importance and collecting and interpreting outcome data on those issues. The processes described for identifying, measuring, and interpreting patient care outcomes are useful for a single patient or for groups of patients. If the idea of conducting outcome studies seems overwhelming, selected skills can be implemented to inform clinical practice immediately without needing to conduct a full outcome study. This book provides examples from the literature of concepts that have been applied in clinical practice that will help the reader appreciate the relevance of the material. Part 2 will help the reader learn the components of an outcome study using documentation from clinical practice. Finally, the links between outcome measurement processes and management for best practice are introduced.

This book will be most useful to those who have had some clinical experience, and an introductory course in research design and statistics. The clinical experience is important for exposure to at least one documentation style, patient management experience, and appreciation of how variations among patients, clinicians, and environments affect patient outcomes. The research design and statistics background is necessary for understanding the ways that data can be analyzed and applied.

THE CLINICIAN AS DATA COLLECTOR

It would be convenient if someone came along and presented PTs with valid and useful outcome data. To that point, there are some very well established and successful researchers, private companies, and funded projects organizing and processing data on behalf of selected institutions, patient groups, and clinicians. These organizations (such as Focus on Therapeutic Outcomes, Inc. and the Uniform Data System for Medical Rehabilitation) should be commended and studied for the groundbreaking work that they have begun; however, a new view of the data collector needs to be nurtured.

This new data collector is an individual PT who has regular contact with patients and who documents the process of service delivery. Each PT can be a change agent for creating documentation formats that support outcome data collection. Each PT is a manager who needs data to reflect on practice and to report to administrators, consumers, and payers. Each PT is a professional who wants to be accountable for clinical decisions in an increasingly autonomous practice environment. This personal commitment to outcome measurement means that each PT is willing to *systematically*, rather than intuitively, evaluate the effectiveness of clinical services. This may seem like a daunting responsibility, but the current circumstances of health-care delivery and reimbursement demand data as the basis for clinical and financial decision making. It is imperative that clinicians learn to routinely document objective patient data as evidence for clinical decisions, and this can happen only if the data are actually collected in a systematic and usable manner.

> *Data are collected from the clinician's documentation.*

Fortunately, the ability to create outcome data is not as difficult as it first seems. There may be skills and terminology to learn, but the essence of creating outcome data may be as simple as learning to translate or reorganize the documentation that has already been collected.

> *Patient data may be recorded, but they might not be useful.*

This book is a guide to a step-by-step process of translation. Skills that are outside the scope of this book, such as using a computer or specific types of software, will not prevent the reader from learning to create, analyze, and interpret a simple data set based on a caseload of patients.

PATIENT CARE MANAGEMENT PARALLELS
THE RESEARCH PROCESS

The process of patient care management involves many different skills, and these skills parallel traditional research processes. Clinicians interview and examine patients, using tests and measures to derive data about the patient's condition. The data help the clinician to develop a hypothesis about the possible causes of the problems that a patient has identified. The clinician uses a combination of clinical experience, patient values and abilities, and current knowledge and literature to choose an intervention to improve the patient's problem. If the patient improves, the assumption is that the intervention was successful. If there is no improvement, the clinician re-evaluates the patient, the assumptions, and the chosen interventions. A new hypothesis drives a change in approach, and the patient is again measured for improvement.

In traditional research, the investigator identifies a question about a condition or situation that needs to be answered. The investigator gathers history about that question by reading literature that might have data related to the question and by interviewing others who have studied the question. The investigator generates a hypothesis to answer the question and then sets up experiments to test the hypothesis. The experiments include selected examinations and tests that generate data that may or may not support the hypothesis. Whether or not the hypothesis is supported, the results spur new hypotheses about the nature of the problem, and additional testing occurs. See Table 1.1.

Table 1.1

The Parallels Between Patient Care and Research	
Patient Care Management Steps	**Traditional Research Steps**
History taking: Interview patients about their problem.	History taking: Read literature and interview other researchers about a question.
Examination: Perform tests and measures to gather objective data about the problem.	Examination: Identify variables and systematically observe phenomena surrounding the question; collect data on responses to tests and measures.
Evaluation: Interpret results of the tests and measures to determine their importance to the patient problem.	Evaluation: Interpret importance of the data from each variable to the question.
Prognosis: Identify the types of changes that can be expected based on the unique types of patient problems.	Prognosis: Identify all the possible answers to the question based on the available data and constraints of the test conditions.
Diagnosis: Identify a condition consistent with the most probable relationship between impairments and resulting functional losses.	Diagnosis: Identify the most probable hypotheses to explain the phenomena surrounding the question.
Intervention: Apply skills and techniques to remedy an impairment or functional limitation.	Intervention: Apply treatments systematically to a variable to study the outcome.
Outcome Measurement: Record objective and subjective data from the patient following intervention about changes in the presenting problem.	Outcome measurement: Measure the variables and phenomena surrounding the question systematically to determine the effect of intervention.

For both the clinician and the researcher, there is a problem that is first identified. Both have ways to collect information to understand the history and complexities of the problem. Both use tests and measures to describe the unique qualities of the problem, and both implement an intervention to test a hypothesis about how to resolve the problem. The parallels between patient management and research underscore that clinicians are already using the skills necessary to produce outcome data and are using that data to inform clinical decision making.

YOU ARE WHAT YOU WRITE

Each patient can be viewed as a research sample of n=1. Each patient presents a unique set of constraints and challenges within which the clinician establishes a need for services, the expected outcomes of services, and the interventions that will achieve the desired results. Documentation on each patient should contain the data to support the management of the patient. To ensure the data are useful, the patient's chart should accurately reflect the clinician's process of patient management, including repeated measurements and clinical decisions.

There is often a discrepancy between what a chart should include and what it *actually* includes. It is important to remember that to an outside reader, if it is not in the chart, it did not happen. This point is critically important. Many therapists say that they consistently measure changes in patient status, and in fact this may be true. Typical problems with clinical measures include that they are:

> *If it is not in the chart, it did not happen.*

- Taken during a patient visit but are not recorded in the patient record for that day.
- Not recorded in the same way each time for the same patient.
- Not recorded at routine intervals, resulting in absent pre- or post-treatment measures.
- Not recorded in the same way across multiple patients, even when the problem is the same.

When charts are systematically reviewed by an outside reader (e.g., an administrator, quality assurance officer, or a peer reviewer), the reviewer may find an absence or inconsistent pattern of information. However, if the type of information collected on similar patients is consistently entered at the same intervals, those measurements become the foundation for a cohort data set.

THE STRENGTH IS IN THE NUMBERS

A cohort data set represents a group of patients who present with the same pathology and signs and symptoms. Although the inclusion and exclusion criteria for each group may differ, the key characteristic of cohort data is that the *same measurements are taken on all the patients at the same points in time* during their episodes of care. Single-case report data can indicate that a strategy is working for an individual patient. In contrast, cohort data show the variability in changes that similar patients will experience from the same intervention strategy as well as the likely effectiveness of a particular intervention. Thus, cohort data are more supportive for predicting outcomes for future patients, whereas single-case data may be more individualized to a patient who is currently receiving care.

> *Measurements taken the same way, at the same points in service, are the building blocks of data sets.*

SOME CHALLENGES OF RETROSPECTIVE CHART REVIEWS

If cohort data provide greater confidence for clinical outcomes and allow for more supported prognoses, why are they not more readily available to clinicians? Quality assurance and health system reviews provide some insight into the challenges of creating cohort data in clinical settings. One challenge is the need to standardize the way measures are taken and recorded within and among clinicians at a single clinical site. This requires achieving agreement on the chosen measures and the manner for documenting those measures from groups of clinicians with different educational backgrounds, skill sets, and preferences. Choosing standardized measures may also cost money for forms and staff training and increase the time spent with a patient; these are costs that may not be perceived as beneficial when weighed against the desire for uniform measures across patients.

Another challenge is that the documentation formats may not be easily converted to usable data sets. Narrative and pencil-and-paper documentation systems cannot support cohort data development as easily or efficiently as scanning or computerized menu-driven systems. The amount of time it takes to transpose data from a subjective, objective, assessment, and plan (SOAP note) to a spreadsheet is considerable and thus is a deterrent to performing retrospective chart reviews.

Small sample sizes limit the generalization of data, but they are still informative. A clinical setting may have usable data on small groups of patients who are served at that clinic, but it may not have enough patients with the same diagnosis to collect data on a group in a reasonable time. Having a way to collect data together with another clinical setting speeds up the number of patients included in a data set but also requires agreement among the clinicians about measurement and documentation methods.

These are just a few of the challenges that clinicians face, but they are not impossible to overcome. This book will explain how to tackle the many challenges to developing cohort data sets from the documentation of a clinician's own case mix.

THE BENEFITS OF CONDUCTING RETROSPECTIVE OUTCOME STUDIES

Despite the difficulties and challenges, there are many reasons to learn the processes of outcome measurement and management. Here are some quotes from clinicians who have conducted small retrospective reviews of their documentation using the processes outlined in the book.

> *"This assessment made me aware of a lot of things I kept on doing that I didn't even realize I was doing."*

> *"Surprising enough is the discovery of the differences in the percentage of functional and impairment goals that were predicted for my data as compared to that of the actual data . . . . It was estimated that functional goals would make up 40% of all the goals set in my data; however, the actual number was calculated as 30%. This does not follow the recommendations of many of the authors . . . ." M. Maione*

> *"My outcomes study has revealed some crucial information on ways to improve customer relations in our facility."* J. Rizzoli

> *"In conclusion, current practice in documenting goals to assess clients with TKA is inconsistent with review of literature on the use of function versus impairment measures and measurability."* L. Pemberton

In all cases, the key benefit to these clinicians was greater knowledge about how to approach their patients. Conducting retrospective outcome studies allows the clinician to view the path traveled, to see the quality and quantity of personal clinical practice, and to make informed decisions as to how to improve. No doubt there is an investment of time for data collection and literature review, but the benefits of a study are multidimensional:

- Updated knowledge about the management or measurement of a particular diagnostic group.
- Data to describe current practice, from which goals for improvement can be developed.
- Objective evidence to guide clinical and managerial decisions.
- Validation that the care provided is consistent with current literature or guidance on bringing practice into alignment with current approaches.
- Improved efficiency and confidence in the ability to look objectively at practice.

HEALTH INSURANCE PORTABILITY AND ACCOUNTABILITY ACT PRIVACY RULE

The Health Insurance Portability and Accountability Act (HIPAA) of 1996 is a federal regulation that protects personal health information (PHI) of patients. The Privacy Rule defines PHI as a patient's demographic, medical, or billing information that is maintained by a service provider or entity (such as hospital) and that could, if revealed, identify the individual patient. The Privacy Rule identifies eight conditions under which materials containing PHI can be used for research, including data sets with deidentification of records. The exercise in this textbook is a retrospective review of records of patients whom the reader has personally treated *and* provided documentation on *and* who has been discharged from services. Development of the data set requires access to medical chart information; however, PHI information is not required for the creation of a deidentified data set and in fact is discouraged for this study. If a clinician is employed by an entity that collects PHI, the clinician may need to seek approval for the study from the institutional review board (IRB) to ensure that the data collection processes meet the IRB requirements. If the clinician is the owner of a practice that maintains medical records, the owner also needs to ensure that the data collection process is consistent with HIPAA requirements. The easiest method for this is a two-step process:

1. Record the data of interest from existing records of discharged patients.
2. Do not record the 18 identifiers as described in the HIPAA regulations. These include:

Name
Geographic information (including city and zip code)
Elements of dates (except year), age over 89 years
Telephone number
Fax number
E-mail address
Social Security number
Medical record, prescription number(s)
Health plan beneficiary/account numbers
Certificate/license number
VIN and serial numbers, license plate number
Device identifiers, serial numbers
Web URLs
IP address
Biometric identifiers (fingerprints)
Full-face, comparable photo images
Unique identifying number(s)

By using a random record number assigned to each patient record, a data set of 10 patients can be compiled for the purposes of the study in this textbook that comply with most "exempt" interpretations of the HIPAA regulations.

The following websites provide information about the HIPAA standards as they relate to research (privacyruleandresearch.nih.gov/healthservicesprivacy.asp) and to IRB responsibilities (privacyruleandresearch.nih.gov/irbandprivacyrule.asp).

SUMMARY

This chapter introduced the reasons for using documentation as a source for data in clinical practice, the parallels between patient management and research processes, and the challenges and benefits of conducting retrospective outcome studies to learn more about practice. Although there are many real challenges to conducting a retrospective study, the clinical and managerial benefits for patients and physical therapy practice can be significant.

References

Delitto A (2005). Research in low back pain: Time to stop seeking the elusive "magic bullet". Physical Therapy 85:206–207.

Duckworth M (1999). Outcome measurement selection and typology. Physiotherapy 85(1):21–27.

Focus on Therapeutic Outcomes, Inc., PO Box 11444, Knoxville, TN 37030 (fotoinc.com).

Haley SM & Jette AM (2000). RRTC for measuring rehabilitation outcomes: Extending the frontier of rehabilitation outcome measurement and research. Journal of Rehabilitation Outcomes Measurement 4(4):31–41.

Jette AM (2005). The peril of inadequate evidence. Physical Therapy 85:302–303.

Keith RA (1998). Patient satisfaction and rehabilitation services. Archives of Physical Medicine and Rehabilitation 79:1122–1128.

Kramer AM (1997). Rehabilitation care and outcomes from the patient's perspective. Medical Care 35(6):JS48–57.

Maione M (2005). Outcome measures for the management of patients with low back pain. Unpublished paper.

McKinley RK, Stevenson K, Adams S, & Manku-Scott TK (2002). Meeting patient expectations of care: The major determinant of satisfaction with out-of-hours primary medical care? Family Practice 19:333–338.

Pemberton L (2005) Total knee replacement outcomes: Type and measurability of goals. Unpublished paper.

Rizzoli J (2005) Outcomes study of charting documentation patterns of patients diagnosed with peripheral vestibular dysfunction. Unpublished paper.

Sackett DL, Strauss SE, Richardson WS, Rosenberg W, & Haynes RB (2000). Evidence-Based Medicine: How to Practice and Teach EBM. Churchill Livingstone, NY.

Seelman KD (2000). Rehabilitation outcomes measurement: State of the art in the year 2000. Journal of Rehabilitation Outcomes Measurement 4(4):1.

Uniform Data System for Medical Rehabilitation, a division of UB Foundation Activities, Inc. 270 Northpointe Parkway, Amherst NY (udsmr.org)

An Outcome Approach to Patient Care Management

KEY TERMS

Health-care outcomes

Therapeutic indicators

Episode of intervention

Patient outcomes

Outcome measures

Fix-it approach

Meaningful result

Evaluate-and-treat approach

Intervention

Outcome approach

Predict and manage

Reflective practitioner

CHAPTER OUTCOMES

➤ Describe an outcome approach to patient care.

➤ Contrast an outcome approach to patient care with other approaches.

An outcome perspective in patient care influences the clinician's approach to patient examination, the organization of documentation, and the expected service outcomes. This chapter introduces a definition of outcomes and relates that definition to patient care management. It describes strategies to use with patients to facilitate an outcome approach to care. Two traditional approaches to patient care are contrasted with an outcome approach. These patient care approaches are related to documentation design. Integration of an outcome approach will help the clinician identify goals that are meaningful to patients and support more efficient paths of intervention to achieve those outcomes.

DEFINING OUTCOMES

The *American Heritage Dictionary* (1981) defines outcome as a "natural result or consequence." Tabor's *Cyclopedic Medical Dictionary* (2005) defines a positive outcome as "the remediation of functional limitation or disability; the prevention of illness or injury; or an improvement in patient satisfaction." This textbook suggests a broader definition of outcomes.

> *Health-care outcomes are meaningful results following an episode of intervention.*

In this book, **health-care outcomes** refer to those categories of measurement or observation that service providers attempt to improve. The observations can be of patients, providers, processes, or entire health-care systems. A single outcome may have a range of results within it. For example, "return to work" is a common patient outcome, with results ranging from "no return to work" to "complete recovery of prior work status." Patient goals are set individually to achieve a selected level of result within a type of outcome. Likewise, administrative goals are selected to achieve a level of result unique to a setting within a category of outcome. Two examples of administrative outcomes are the cost of service and the level of patient satisfaction.

Outcome measures refer to tools or procedures used to quantify progress toward an expected outcome. These tools may be published evaluations that produce a score or measurement strategies that are reproducible across clinicians, patients, or administrators. Examples of measurement tools include the Barthel Index and the SF-36; examples of measurement strategies include the Timed-Up-and-Go and the calculation of gait velocity.

Ideally, in patient care, a **meaningful result** is one that has relevance to at least two people or parties: the patient receiving the service and the service provider. Although it is possible to argue that an outcome can be meaningful to just one party, strategies for achieving outcomes are enhanced by mutual cooperation. In addition to the patient and the provider, other parties may have an interest in the results. These parties include family members, referral sources, other health-care providers who are working with the same patient, service administrators, and researchers.

An **episode of intervention** is defined as those activities that occur within a specified time. In physical therapy, the expectation is that the activities are purposeful and goal-directed. In administrative studies, the activities may be related to policy changes or service changes. The time frame for an episode of patient intervention may be a single session or a series of sessions. The time frame for administrative interventions might be a fiscal quarter, a year, or decades. An episode of intervention is operationally defined as all the patient management or service activities that occur between the initial and final follow-up measures; those measurement points are determined by the person measuring the outcomes. The time frame for patients may be immediately before and after a single session of care, a series of sessions, or from baseline to some time following discharge from services. In longitudinal outcome studies, the time frame for the follow-up measures might be years or decades.

The **intervention** is defined as those activities performed in the delivery of service. In rehabilitation, it most often refers to activities used by the clinician to advance the patient toward the goals. The activities might include a single intervention or series of interventions that a patient receives directly from a clinician, such as learning a home exercise program, performing a series of joint mobilizations, or participating in a cardiac rehabilitation program. Administrators might look at activities that a patient must do in order to receive services, such as making an appointment and completing intake procedures, or, at larger service processes, such as billing or interdepartmental coordination.

Examples of the Definition Applied to Studies

The study by Arnetz, et al. (2004) can be used to illustrate the definition that *Health-care outcomes are meaningful results following an episode of intervention.*

   Title. Active patient involvement in the establishment of physical therapy goals: effects on treatment outcomes and quality of care.

   Health-care outcomes. Patients completed a questionnaire about expectations of care and current health status.

   Meaningful results. The intervention group had statistically higher levels of goal achievement, impairment changes, and perceptions of quality of care.

   Episode of intervention. 10 months of service provision at a rheumatology clinic.

   Intervention. Two randomized groups of patients received either traditional physical therapy or a combination of traditional therapy and participation in a "goal forum" during which the patient and the clinician compared expected treatment goals for improvement of impairments, activities of daily living limitations, and basic functional mobility skills.

The study by Arnetz, et al. (2004) demonstrates both the clinical and managerial perspectives in a single study. Patients who participated in the goal forum had better clinical outcomes, and the overall perception of the quality of care they received was higher, which is an important outcome to the management.

A study by Binder, et al. (2004) illustrates the definition of outcomes for a patient-oriented study on hip fracture rehabilitation.

   Health-care outcomes. Improved functional status and perceived quality of life post hip fracture.

   Meaningful results. Patients receiving extended physical therapy achieved higher physical performance test and functional status questionnaire scores and greater strength, walking speed, and balance than those receiving home exercise programs.

Episode of intervention. Six months with a baseline measure, and repeated measures at 3 and 6 months.

Interventions. Community-dwelling elders post hip fracture repair were randomized into a typical home exercise program group or an extended outpatient physical therapy group with progressive resistive exercise.

From these examples, the definition of outcomes is useful at the patient level and at a broader service level. This text will focus primarily on the measurement of patient-related outcomes, but the processes can easily be applied to management outcomes.

AN OUTCOME APPROACH TO PATIENT CARE

The outcome approach to physical therapy patient care can be summarized as "predict and manage," where the result of care or the *outcome* is predicted before intervention begins, and the clinician manages the available resources and interventions toward achieving the goal. An outcome approach to patient care begins with identifying the endpoint of care in collaboration with the patient. The functional limitations or losses that are important to the patient need to be determined in order to set meaningful goals for care. Once the goals are set, the criteria for achieving them can be determined so both the patient and physical therapist (PT) know when to end care. Clear goals with measurable characteristics provide the basis for choosing interventions to achieve the goals. The outcome approach to patient care requires good interviewing skills, an understanding of expected outcomes for a variety of diagnoses, and the creativity to identify how the unique needs or wishes of a patient can be realized through intervention.

A Travel Analogy

➤ *Both travelers and patients need answers to "Where are we going?" and "Why are we going there?"*

The outcome approach to patient care is analogous to two people who want to travel together. First, the travelers must decide where they are going and why that destination is important. These answers give direction to the journey. The travelers may have very different ideas about where to go on this trip: one may want a quiet, sunny beach, but the other may want the hustle and bustle of a busy city. In order for the two travelers to agree on a destination, they will need to share their expectations and then choose one of four options.

OPTION 1: One person's goal takes precedence over the other. This usually results in at least one satisfied traveler, and possibly two.

OPTION 2: Compromise. Each gets a little of what each wants, but both let go of some goals. This can result in two moderately satisfied travelers.

OPTION 3: Find a destination that meets both their needs. This results in two satisfied travelers.

OPTION 4: Postpone traveling together. Either more information is needed to make a decision, or each traveler goes a separate way with the option to travel together at a future time.

Determining Patient Care Goals With an Outcome Approach

The PT and the patient are similar to the travelers. Together, the PT and the patient need to determine a meaningful functional outcome before intervention strategies can be selected to achieve the outcome. As with the travelers, the result of the initial encounter can proceed in four ways.

OPTION 1: One person's goal may take precedence. If the PT sets the goal for the patient, it's possible that the patient will not agree with or be satisfied with the outcome. If the patient sets the goal, the PT may not feel it is reasonably attainable.

OPTION 2: Compromise. Both the patient and the PT set reasonable goals. If the patient compromises on goals that are personally very important, the patient may feel dissatisfied at the end of service despite the achievement of the agreed-upon goals. If the PT compromises on goals, there may be concerns about injury recurrence.

OPTION 3: Identify the same goals as priorities. In this case, both the PT and the patient are the most satisfied because there is agreement about the goals, and the criteria for ending care are clear.

OPTION 4: Delay the start of care. This may occur because the goals are too discrepant or because there is not enough information about the expected outcomes to accept any of the options.

The outcomes to which the patient and PT agree will need to be well defined in terms of the patient's needs, the living and work environments, the resources available, and the medical prognosis for functional recovery. Once the PT and the patient agree on the outcomes, they can move forward with determining how to achieve them.

This approach to patient care is consistent with the Hypothesis-Oriented Algorithm for Clinicians II (HOAC II) as described by Rothstein, Echternach, and Riddle (2003). In this model of clinical decision making, the starting point is the patient-identified problem, which is "almost exclusively descriptions of functional limitations and disabilities" (Rothstein, Echternach, & Riddle, 2003, p. 459) (Fig. 2.1).

Patient Outcomes Are Different From Therapeutic Indicators

One of the more confusing distinctions to appreciate in an outcome approach to patient management is the difference between patient outcomes and therapeutic indicators about the effectiveness of intervention. In other words, it is necessary to distinguish the difference between the patient's functional goals and the therapist's impairment indicators. Physical therapy documentation should include patient goals that are meaningful to the patient; these are the patient outcomes. The goals will focus on improving function, preferably in the contexts in which the functions should happen, because this is what is important to the patient. Subsequent documentation should report measures of the functional goals to indicate a change in patient status.

➤ Patient goals reflect function; impairments are therapy indicators for the clinician.

Measures of impairment are generally more meaningful to the PT than to the patient. Changes in impairments indicate that a change at the tissue level is occurring, whether related to the intervention, time to heal, or some other factor. If the clinical hypothesis is that function will improve as

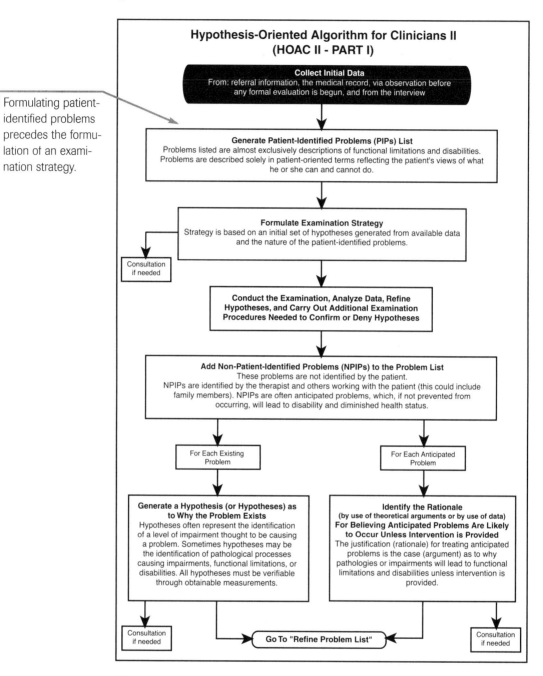

Formulating patient-identified problems precedes the formulation of an examination strategy.

Figure 2.1 Hypothesis-Oriented Algorithm for Clinicians II. (From Rothstein JM, Echternach JL & Riddle DL [2003]. The Hypothesis Oriented Algorithm for Clinicians II [HOAC II]: A guide for patient management. Physical Therapy 83:455–470)

impairments are reduced, then interventions will be aimed at the impairments. Reduction of impairments suggests that the chosen interventions are having an impact, but the ultimate test of the clinical hypothesis is whether the functional status improves. It is important to document changes in impairment status in the patient record, and these measures are useful for outcome studies of intervention effectiveness, but changes in impairments should not be the patient's goals. Objective performance measures of functional goals help the patient to recognize that therapy is working and put achievement of the targeted behavior in the real-life context in which it needs to happen. For example, strengthening (the intervention) may reduce lower extremity weakness as determined by a dynamometer (the impairment measure), but an increase in several pounds of pressure is not as relevant to the patient as whether the patient can now ascend steps (the functional outcome) at home (the context). A patient may understand and be able to describe many of his or her own impairments; however, the reason the patient seeks physical therapy is because of the loss in function, not just the presence of impairments. Even when pain is the predominant impairment, patients seek help because the pain interferes with comfortable or efficient function.

Most therapists would say that they are working on functional goals for the patient, and most likely they are. The issue here is whether the *documentation* does or does not reflect measures of the functional goals for the patient. In an outcome approach, the patient goals should reflect the desired functional gains, and documentation should include repeated measures of functional changes. Documentation on impairments serves as support for clinical decision making about how to achieve the functional goals but are not the ultimate patient outcomes.

Linking measures of impairments to measures of functional change is consistent with the step of "establishing testing criteria" in the HOAC II (Rothstein, Echternach, & Riddle, 2003). In this step, measures of change often relate to the impairments that are hypothesized to be related to the functional limitation, but changes in impairments are intervention goals, not patient goals.

Selecting Interventions

Once the clinician and the patient agree on the outcomes of care, interventions need to be selected to achieve the goals. Many factors influence the selection process, most notably time and money. A short time frame and a distant goal may require a highly intensive approach, whereas a long time frame might allow for a less intensive approach. Consider the professional athlete who needs an intensive rehabilitation approach because her livelihood or athletic rating depends on getting back into competition very quickly. Contrast that with the recreational athlete who prefers a less aggressive, more gradual approach because the priorities of work, family, and other responsibilities limit the time and resources that can be spent each day or week on a rehabilitation program.

> *For travelers and patients, strategies to achieve the goal are influenced by many variables.*

Using a clinical hypothesis to express the relationship between the patient's *current* status and the *desired* level of function is a helpful step in selecting interventions. The variables that limit function most often include physical impairments but may also include environmental factors, patient resources and motivation, and even the therapist's resources and skills. During an initial examination, many clinical abnormalities or limitations might be identified. The key is to identify which cluster of the many findings, if corrected, will allow the patient to achieve the goals. A clearly articulated hypothesis identifies the relationship between impairments and environmental factors and the functional losses. Several hypotheses might be generated for a single patient outcome, but one will need to be acted on first. The choice may be influenced by prior clinical experience, by current literature, or by

> *Clinical hypotheses should drive the selection of interventions.*

the patient's unique situation. In the end, one hypothesis will be selected on which to start a plan of care. If the patient improves as a result of the care, then the hypothesis is supported. If the patient does *not* improve after a couple of visits, a re-examination of the situation might lead to the selection of a different hypothesis and a change in interventions.

Consider the following clinical example. A coal miner was complaining of unilateral carpal tunnel symptoms because it was interfering with his work of shoveling coal onto coal cars. The patient's goal was to be able to work a full shift each day shoveling coal. Hypothesis 1 addresses the impairments caused by tissue irritation, and the selected interventions are aimed at relieving the tissue irritation to allow the patient to work with fewer interruptions.

HYPOTHESIS 1 ■ Shoveling coal for 8 hours causes tissue irritation across the wrist, which leads to inflammation that causes nerve impingement. The resulting numbness, pain, and weakness in the patient's hand require unacceptably frequent interruptions in shoveling.

Selected Intervention: Intervention to reduce inflammation should relieve the impingement and reverse the symptoms, so a regimen of icing, gentle stretching, and soft-tissue mobilization is selected. A soft splint is provided to wear between shifts to protect the wrist from additional aggravation. Therapy is recommended three times a week for the first week and twice weekly thereafter until symptoms are relieved.

Although this hypothesis seems reasonable, it only addresses the impact of the impairments on the goal. A hypothesis that addresses a combination of factors will drive a different selection of interventions. In Hypothesis 2, tissue irritation is the impairment, and ergonomic characteristics of shoveling on a coal line are also addressed.

HYPOTHESIS 2 ■ Excessive shoveling on one side of the coal line causes tissue irritation across the wrist, which leads to inflammation that causes nerve impingement. The resulting numbness, tingling, and weakness in the patient's hand require unacceptably frequent interruptions in shoveling.

Selected Intervention: Prevention of overuse at the wrist should reduce the cause of irritation, so the patient is educated to alternate the sides of the coal line on which the patient shovels coal and to do periodic stretches during shift breaks to reduce future symptoms. Four clinic visits are recommended to address the acute inflammation with icing, gentle stretching, and soft-tissue mobilization.

In Hypothesis 2, both the impairments and the ergonomic variables are addressed so that the plan of care is more inclusive and requires fewer visits by the patient. In fact, in this example adapted from actual practice, the therapist acted on Hypothesis 2. The coal miner merely had to switch sides with a partner at regular intervals to use the opposite shoveling pattern. The symptoms were relieved, and the coal miner could maintain full employment.

In summary, an outcome approach to patient care management requires setting a goal that is meaningful and reasonable to the patient as well as to the therapist. Based on the goal, the therapist can derive a clinical hypothesis that relates the patient's presentation to the desired goal. The clinical hypothesis influences the selection of intervention strategies for meeting the goals while recognizing time and budget constraints.

ALL OUTCOMES ARE RELATIVE

Health services outcomes encompass a wide variety of measures. The same outcome in one setting may be important to that setting and of little interest in another. In other words, there is no consensus on what should be measured, except that the measures should be important to the parties involved.

Health service and patient outcomes are linked to the unique environment in which they occur and are influenced by many factors. The differences may be the result of the type of intervention provided (Indredavik, et al., 1998), the intensity of treatment sessions (Jette, Warren, & Wirtalla, 2005), the socioeconomic and cultural values that patients bring to the rehabilitation process (Cook, et al., 2005), or the family structure and support (Jia, et al., 2005), to name a few. For example, in a landmark study, Wennberg and Gittelsohn (1982) demonstrated that the type and amount of care patients receive depended on geographic location and local medical practice patterns. Indredavik, et al. (1998) demonstrated that patients who were discharged to specialized stroke rehabilitation units had better quality of life outcomes 5 years after discharge as compared with patients who received rehabilitation through a local general hospital. Figure 2.2 depicts some of the factors that affect the outcomes of intervention. When interpreting outcome data for a single patient, a group of patients, or an entire health service organization, it is important to recognize the impact that these factors may have on the outcome of interest.

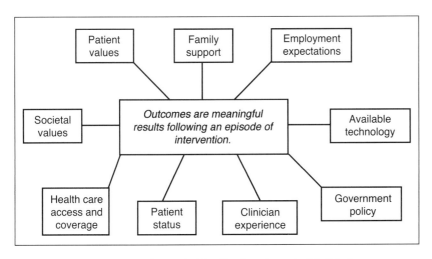

Figure 2.2 Factors impacting on the identification of meaningful clinical outcomes.

STRATEGIES FOR ENSURING SATISFACTION WITH THE GOALS

Patients and clinicians both want positive results from an episode of care; both want the patients to achieve their goals. Patients who keep their appointments are making a commitment of time and money to address an important functional loss. There is nothing more frustrating for a patient than to receive treatments for a problem and to see no evidence that the problem is resolving. From the PT's perspective, when patients discontinue therapy before the expected outcomes are achieved, the PT wonders why the services were not valued. There are number of strategies that a clinician can use during patient encounters to increase the likelihood of achieving satisfaction with the outcomes of care.

Begin at the End

In almost all cases, goals are meaningful to a patient if the goals are focused on the recovery of function (Randall & McEwen, 2000) rather than on the changing of impairment status. Goals that are valued by the patient directly influence the choice of tests and measures and interventions. For example, the ability to climb steps at home or work will be more relevant to a patient than the number of pounds lifted during a straight leg raise. While the strengthening of the leg may be needed to climb stairs, the improved strength ratings are not meaningful to a patient if function does not change as well.

To identify the patient's goals, the clinician should ask questions that help the patient focus on the activities or skills that have been lost as a result of the most immediate condition (Box 2.1). This process is especially important for patients with chronic conditions because repeated episodes of care will probably address different goals. The clinician needs to identify how the scale tipped for a person who may have been:

- Healthy but sustained an injury.
- Tolerating a certain amount of discomfort or functional compromise but has experienced a meaningful reduction in function.
- Tolerating an impairment but now wants to alter its impact on quality of life or social opportunity.

BOX 2.1

Sample Questions to Begin a Patient Interview

- "What do you hope to achieve by receiving physical therapy?"
- "How do you want physical therapy to help you?"
- "What activities are harder to perform as a result of your condition?"
- "Which ones are most important for you to regain?"
- "How will you know you are better?"
- "What and/or how much change in function will you need to end treatment?"

By focusing on a change in status or a change in the need to perform tasks more efficiently, the patient has tipped the personal scale from that of compromising to that of seeking help.

Going back to the travel analogy, this is the part of the patient-clinician dialogue where a vision of the destination is described. These questions put the responsibility on the patient to become an active partner in the rehabilitation process. When a patient can clearly identify what the goal is and the value of performing that task, the patient will be able to recognize when the goal is met. Think about a personal travel experience. Recall the stress of taking a train or bus ride and not knowing when to get off because the landmarks were not recognizable or the signs were in a different language. When there is a clear picture of the destination, it is easier to determine if one has arrived.

Include the Patient in Goal Setting

Including the patient when setting goals improves patient compliance (Bassett & Petrie, 1999; Friedrich, et al., 1998), improves clinical outcomes (Arnetz, et al., 2004), and clarifies expectations to reduce unmet goals (Bell, et al., 2002). One patient may have very clear and reasonable goals for functional change. Another patient may not know why he was referred to physical therapy or what improvement to expect as a result of intervention. With a guided interview and some direct questions, a patient will be able to tell the clinician how life activities have been limited as well as the importance of regaining those activities. When a patient clarifies which functional losses are most important, the foundation for meaningful goals is in place.

Including the patient in setting goals improves the odds that the patient will understand the purpose of the interventions and be more invested in the physical therapy outcomes (Bassett & Petrie, 1999). When the PT assumes sole responsibility for determining the goals, the patient is allowed to begin the episode of care without having to take responsibility for the rehabilitation process. That may be initially comforting for the less experienced patient, but it sets the expectation that the PT will manage care *for*, rather than *with*, the patient. For the patient with a chronic condition, who has had multiple experiences with physical therapy, there may already be expectations for the outcomes of services (Arnetz, et al., 2004).

When economic constraints limit the visits that a patient can afford, establishing an active partnership with the patient is essential for achieving the goals efficiently and economically.

Even when the patient is a passive recipient of care, the patient may have outcome expectations. If the patient expectations match those of the clinician, then the therapy experience may, *coincidentally*, be quite satisfactory. If the expectations are different, whether or not the clinician is aware of that difference, the therapy experience may not be as positive. The patient may not understand the purpose of the interventions, may have different expectations of change, may not comply with home programs that seemingly have no relationship to the patient's goals, or may not voice his or her real concerns during an initial examination. When a patient lacks ownership of the goals, there is greater likelihood that the patient may not comply with intervention (Bell, et al., 2002), that status changes may not be understood by the patient, and that overall satisfaction with the service will be low (Kaplan,

Greenfield, & Ware, 1989; Starfield, et al., 1981). Patients make decisions about returning for subsequent treatment based in part on the quality of the interpersonal relationship experienced in the first encounter, the patient's belief that the clinician listened, and if the patient perceived being included in the decision-making process (Grimmer, et al., 1999). It is easier for patients who do not see the value of the goal or who do not understand the intervention experience to cancel, not show for appointments, or discontinue coming altogether.

When functional goals are meaningful to the patient, participation in the rehabilitation process is enhanced. The patient's role in the evaluation of change becomes more active. The patients are better reporters about changes that occur outside the clinic and better monitors of their response to treatment because the goals are related to tasks that have personal meaning. Thus, one essential component of the initial patient interview should be determining meaningful and achievable patient goals.

Ask Direct Questions

It may help to begin the initial patient encounter by asking very direct questions about the patient's expectations (see Box 2.1). Beginning an examination with direct questions allows the clinician to establish the patient's knowledge of his or her condition and whether specific goals exist. For the patient who does have goals, these direct questions will help determine how reasonable the goals are and what motivates the patient.

Therapists may have concerns that patients do not know what physical therapy can do for them; however, patients indicate that they feel prepared to collaborate in goal setting (Baker, et al., 2001). For many patients, the referral may be the first time they have heard of the profession; for them, direct questions become even more important because the questions can help them learn what types of problems can and cannot be addressed by physical therapy. Regardless of the patient's knowledge of physical therapy, a patient does understand the extent of functional loss that has resulted from an injury or disease and whether he or she needs or wants to recover those functions. The challenge for the clinician is to choose the right questions to ask.

Identify the Value Placed by the Patient on Functional Losses

Direct questions about loss of function help patients articulate their own unique functional losses and the relative importance of those losses. It is easy to assume that patients with the same diagnosis and classic presentation of impairments might also have similar goals. In fact, for many medical diagnoses, there are goals that most patients share. For example, it is expected that patients who were walking before a total hip replacement will have a goal for walking after surgery. While the classic presentation is critical for the therapist to use as a foundation for the examination of the patient, not all patients will have the same presentation, and not all the typical functional limitations will be equally important to all patients. An example of this is commonly seen with patients who have had a stroke. Independent walking skills may be a high priority for some patients, whereas the use of walker may be preferred by others. Some patients may see choosing a walker as a decline in function or a less normal mode of mobility, and others will consider the walker as a desirable and effective means for improving function because they can keep up with their peers and feel more secure.

Identifying the right goal for each patient requires that the clinician distinguish between what *can* be accomplished from what the patient *wants* to accomplish. It requires a depth of probing and patient interviewing for which some therapists may feel unprepared (Baker, et al., 2001). Sometimes the patient's expectations of rehabilitation are too high, unrealistic based on the prognosis of the medical condition, or just different (Bradley, et al., 2000). In these situations, the clinician and the patient must continue the dialogue in order to reach agreement on what can be achieved. Baker, et al. (2001) found that in 50% of initial examinations, there were no explicit statements about what the final goals of therapy would be, even though the therapists had strong beliefs that collaboration on the goals is important. Campbell, Quilty, and Dieppe (2003) found that answers on standardized questionnaires completed by patients were discrepant with answers obtained through interviews (Table 2.1). Whether goal setting occurs implicitly during the examination process or therapists feel pressured by time constraints, the final goals of therapy may not be consistently communicated or clarified with the patient. When the patient clearly understands the goals of therapy and the reasons for the selected interventions, compliance is enhanced (Friedrich, et al., 1998).

Educate the Patient

When the patient is unable to identify how function should improve or has unrealistic expectations, the clinician is responsible for educating the patient. During the initial examination, the clinician can help the patient articulate

Table 2.1

Comparison of Questionnaire vs. Interview Responses on Change in Status				
	QUESTIONNAIRE			
Interview	Better	No change	Worse	Total
Pain scores				
Better	6	1	2	9
No change	7	2	1	10
Worse	1	0	0	1
Total	14	3	3	20*
Disability scores				
Better	3	4	4	11
No change	3	2	3	8
Worse	1	0	0	1
Total	7	6	7	20*

*6 men and 14 women: 6 were age 45-59 years, 5 were age 60-69 years, and 9 were age 70 years or older. From Campbell R, Quilty B & Dieppe P. (2003). Discrepancies between patient's assessments of outcome: qualitative study nested within a randomized controlled trial. British Medical Journal 326: 252–253.

how a medical condition has affected their daily function and role requirements. Other factors may modify the goals or the interventions, but the starting point for intervention is always the predicted outcome that is relevant to the patient's need for function.

When the patient is not able to describe functional losses or cannot identify what an improvement would be, the patient may not be ready to benefit from intervention, and the therapist may not be able to intervene effectively. After all, if the patient does not know where she is going, how will she know when she gets there? The patient needs to know which "destinations" or milestones will be achieved as a result of intervention. The PT needs to look for these same milestones to know when to discharge the patient. Ideally, in an outcome approach, *the clinician and the patient agree on discharge criteria in the first visit before treatment begins.*

Patients who cannot identify the changes they would like to see as a result of intervention may need time to reflect on or observe their limitations. These patients may benefit from keeping a journal about what they can and cannot do during the course of a single day or week in order to identify how activities are limited. A journal helps the patient identify goals that have direct relevance to the patient's daily life and environments in which the patient functions. With this clarity about functional limitations, the patient can better negotiate meaningful outcomes with a PT and thus improve the likelihood of success and satisfaction.

Identify Meaningful Measures of Functional Change

It can be very frustrating to hear a teacher say, "You're getting better, but you need more practice." Vague feedback about a developing skill does not allow the student to identify how progress is measured. When a patient knows how to measure or observe functional changes, the patient becomes better focused on the goals of intervention and on the reporting of pertinent information. Patients who are capable of counting the repetitions completed in their home exercise programs are also capable of counting the laps walked between rooms in their homes, the time it takes to get dressed, and the number of times someone assists them during bathing. Emphasizing measurement of functional activities keeps the patient and the clinician focused on meaningful changes.

Converting functional activities into measurable goals can be a challenge because the conditions for performance are not always the same. Task analysis is a useful process for developing an objective measure of task completion. By guiding a patient through the task and listing the steps from beginning to end, the clinician can derive a measure of independent completion. The patient can check off the steps completed independently at home and bring the chart to therapy sessions. As impairments resolve or the use of adaptive equipment becomes easier, the patient should be able to complete more steps independently. Once the patient can do all the steps of the task, speed, accuracy, or endurance can be measured until the functional goals are met. The improved performance noted on the task analysis is motivating for many patients because they continually review their goals and see progress. This specific strategy of feedback about their functional progress may enhance compliance with both home programs and clinic visits because the goals remain meaningful.

AN OUTCOME APPROACH TO EXAMINATION IS DIFFERENT

There are two approaches to service delivery that have existed comfortably in health-care systems. Lynn and DeGrazia (1991) called one the **fix-it** approach, and the other will be referred to as the **evaluate-and-treat** approach. Both approaches have been useful in the evolution of rehabilitation service delivery. The **outcome** approach can be viewed as the next phase in the evolution of rehabilitation service delivery.

The Fix-It Approach

The fix-it approach to health care is a stereotype of practice where the focus of care is on curing, alleviating, or modifying patient problems and using normal health as the standard of comparison (Lynn & DeGrazia, 1991). The patient-clinician interaction is unidirectional, with the patient presenting the problems and the clinician suggesting treatments to alleviate them. This approach does not include a specified time limit for intervention; restoration to normal varies, depending on the initial level of severity. Care continues until normality is restored. The fix-it approach has been an acceptable paradigm in medicine, especially as many acute diagnoses can be fully cured. Rehabilitation services have grown out of the medical model and, by association, have adopted the desire to restore patients to normal levels when it is physiologically or anatomically possible. While this is an admirable goal, it is often not feasible or possible to restore patients to a normal standard, and it is under these circumstances that the fix-it approach no longer works.

The outcome approach is different from the fix-it approach in several ways. It does not necessarily look to restore normal physiological and anatomical function as its primary focus. In contrast, the outcome approach emphasizes measurable changes in function that use the patient's perspective to judge the appropriateness of the outcome (Lynn & DeGrazia, 1991). In other words, all outcomes are relative to the patient's needs, not relative to a normal standard. An outcome approach also specifies a time limit for care (Lynn & DeGrazia, 1991). Although the outcome approach would not rule out returning someone to normal status, the focus is on maximizing function within a given period or episode of care. Estimates of what can be realistically achieved in a given period are directly linked to the interventions that can efficiently and effectively achieve the goal.

The Evaluate-and-Treat Approach

The evaluate-and-treat approach is observed more often in rehabilitation settings than in primary medical care settings. This approach begins with establishing a list of impairments during the initial examination. The emphasis is on identifying deviations from normal movement or sensory patterns and then linking these deviations to interventions that can address them. Goals are based on a general sense of which deviations can be remedied, which in turn will improve the status of the patient. The process of identification of deviations and interventions is often unidirectional, with the clinician advising the patient about the changes that can be made in his or her condition. Time limits for interventions do not necessarily influence which deviations are addressed or whether alternate outcomes ought to be pursued. The success of treatment is measured by improvements in any or all impairments or deviations as they approach the normal standards.

The outcome approach is different from the evaluate-and-treat approach primarily in its starting point. The outcome approach starts with the patient's functional limitations; that is, it starts with activity performance, not impairments. The examination processes unfold to identify the impairments or deviations that might be limiting the functional losses, rather than identifying all impairments or deviations present. In an outcome approach, other impairments may exist, but if they do not appear related to the patient's functional losses, they need not be addressed in the intervention plan.

> *In an outcome approach, only selected impairments may be addressed.*

The evaluate-and-treat approach has been evident in physical therapy service delivery for a long time and may have its origins in three areas. The first may be in the physical therapy educational process. Much of the educational experience is necessarily spent learning about what is normal, what is abnormal or impaired, the indications and contraindications of interventions, and the matching of interventions to alleviate abnormalities or impairments. This process of identifying correct and complete lists of impairments is carried forth and rewarded in early clinical experiences. In a sense, impairment measures became the equivalent of medical laboratory values in that normal standards can be clearly identified. From an educational standpoint, this has been a reasonable teaching plan because it emphasizes foundational knowledge, and learning can be measured objectively based on what is identified correctly. A reciprocal process of linking impairments to functional losses occurs gradually in professional education, with reinforcement assumed to occur during clinical experiences. Changes in educational curricula that emphasize problem-based learning, outcome measurement, and evidenced-based practice have moved clinicians toward an outcome perspective; however, if documentation systems do not reflect the shift from impairments to function in the clinic, then thought processes and examination processes often revert back to an impairment-oriented, evaluate-and-treat approach.

The evolution of professional autonomy has also emphasized the evaluate-and-treat model. Rehabilitation specialties have grown out of the medical model and have had to emerge from under the direction of medical profession as greater autonomy has been sought. It has been the mark of professional respect to receive physician referrals that read "evaluate and treat." In contrast, it is considered an affront to the clinician's knowledge and decision-making skills to receive a referral that dictates a particular formula for treatment or a setting for a prescribed modality. In the effort to gain autonomy, PTs have become experts in quantifying and documenting impairments, sometimes at the expense of quantifying and documenting functional limitations.

Whereas improvement in functional status has always been at the heart of rehabilitation service, it has not always been the focus of research efforts. From the late 1970s through the mid-1990s, there were large advances in technology and computer-based measurement devices. The desire for measurement precision and reliability naturally had researchers focused on measuring impairments rather than functional tasks. Changes in functional status and methods of measuring function were less frequently studied, based in part on the prevalent assumption that changes in impairments would automatically result in the desired changes in function (Jette, 1995). Clinical practice, reinforced by third party payment practices, put a high value on impairment measurement accuracy as well. Emphasis on the measurement of function and measurement of the relationship between impairment changes and functional changes have only recently become the focus of research efforts. Regardless of what has occurred in the past, changes in consumer expectations of accountability require an outcome approach.

DOCUMENTATION FORMATS AND THE OUTCOME APPROACH

Health policy and reimbursement trends have shifted from accepting changes in impairment status as appropriate patient goals to expecting evidence of improved functional abilities (Johnston & Granger, 1994). Documentation of functional goals for the patient will improve the therapist's compliance with health policy and reimbursement expectations (Randall & McEwen, 2000). If documentation is to reflect an outcome approach, the clinician needs to consider the location of the patient goals, when the goals are written, and what happens after they are recorded.

Location of the Goals

Throughout this chapter, identifying the patient's goals for therapy at the beginning of the first encounter has been stressed. It logically follows that the documentation should have a place at the beginning of the form to record the patient's goals. In fact, many documentation forms do not have the patient goals at the beginning, but rather at the end, of the form. Typically, there is room to record past medical history and the results of tests and measures before a place appears to record patient goals. These forms parallel the evaluate-and-treat process; that is, documentation of the abnormalities occurs first, regardless of their relationship to and before determining which goals to focus on (see Appendix 2A).

When the documentation follows an outcome approach, the place to record the patient's goals will be located early in the document. The goals become an anchor on which to report the results of related tests and measures, and the clinical hypotheses reflect the evaluation of the importance of selected test results. The CMS 700 (see Appendix 2B) is an example of how the layout of the document parallels an outcome approach. The goals are identified first, and then the test and measures related to the goals are documented.

Patient Exposure to the Goals

In addition to documenting the patient goals early in the paperwork flow, it helps to identify how the patient finds out about the goals that are written there. In many clinical scenarios, the PT writes up the initial encounter after the patient has left the department. When this happens, the goals may be discussed with the patient during the treatment session, but the final goals documented in the medical record are the ones that the therapist chooses to write about. They may or may not fully reflect the values and desires of the patient, or they may not have been clearly identified for the patient.

In some clinical settings, the patient needs to initial or sign the goals before leaving the initial appointment. This type of process increases the likelihood that the patient understands and agrees with the goals of treatment, but it is not a guarantee. A patient may sign off on goals but not really under-stand them, depending on the amount of jargon and abbreviations used. The power of the traditional clinician-patient relationship may also leave the patient feeling intimidated, so questions or disagreements are limited if the patient thinks they will compromise the care received. In an outcome approach, extra care is taken to ensure that the patient knows what the goals of intervention are and how change will be measured so that both the patient and the clinician are focused on the same measures of change and the same criteria for ending care.

REFLECTIVE PRACTICE AND SELF-EVALUATION

This chapter has described the outcome perspective and its application to managing the individual patient. The focus of discussion has been on the real-time encounter with one patient; that is, when a patient is with the cli-nician in the clinical setting. Ultimately, a clinician should be able to identify a level of effectiveness in achieving the goals that have been set within selected groups of patients. As practice evolves and interventions can be applied with greater dosing accuracy, the clinician should expect to see improved levels of effectiveness. However, the ability to measure practice effectiveness is possible only if the clinician reflects on practice and measures patient outcomes.

The reflective practitioner is someone who continually evaluates his or her effectiveness as a PT (Tichenor & Davidson, 1997). Many therapists believe that patient participation in therapy is important (Baker, et al., 2001), and many clinicians have an intuitive sense of their performance consistency during examinations, but if asked for data to support that intuitive estimate, they are often at a loss. In fact, the forward momentum in a busy department encourages a cycle of documenting patient status in the present, on the day seen, without time or mechanisms to look back over a history of similar patients. Given the climate of increased accountability for health-care dollars and services, clinicians should be thinking of methods to organize daily doc-umentation to allow for retrospective outcome studies.

The first step in that process is to look at the organization and quality of the existing documentation process. Documentation formats that include categorical descriptors, lists of conditions to check off, and fields for infor-mation that remind the clinician to ask specific questions will encourage greater standardization of data than narrative notes. However, just having the fields on a form does not ensure that the information will be included or, if documented, that it will appear in the same manner for all patients. Thus, a common problem with evaluating clinical effectiveness is that the data are not easy to summarize. The purpose of this book is to take a clinician through the steps of distilling data from the clinical documentation already collected. Learning the steps for converting clinical documentation into use-ful data provides a basic skill set for analyzing clinical practice patterns and provides a starting point from which to refine clinical outcomes.

At the end of this chapter, there is a documentation analysis exercise designed to identify the characteristics of the documentation process that the clinician uses. This exercise is a critical starting point for any clinician who is interested in performing outcome studies. If the documentation processes do not lend themselves to collecting quantitative data, then the clinic may need to address documentation practices prior to conducting any studies.

Students and clinicians can use this analysis to evaluate the layout of any initial evaluation form, whether from clinical experiences or forms available on the Web or samples of forms in this chapter.

SUMMARY

Changing health-care delivery systems are demanding greater accountability for the outcomes of intervention such that clinicians must now predict outcomes and manage patients toward them within a set time. Previous models of rehabilitation service delivery were effective for their time. The evolution of rehabilitation service delivery now requires a model that emphasizes accountability to patients as the consumers of interventions and for the intervention processes used by PTs.

The outcome approach to patient care in physical therapy begins with the end in mind. Both the clinician and the patient mutually agree on the outcomes of care. Intervention services are provided after identifying the amount of measurable or observable change in function that will mark the end of services. The outcome approach can be applied to management of the individual patient or to management of entire service delivery systems. In either case, the expected outcome is based on information gathered from the patient or the system, and intervention plans are considered that take unique environmental and consumer constraints into account. With greater focus on accountability, it is important to become reflective of clinical practice and to develop mechanisms for measuring clinical outcomes.

References

American Heritage Dictionary (1981). Houghton Mifflin Company, Boston.

Arnetz JE, Almin I, Bergstrom K, Franzen Y, & Nilsson H (2004). Active patient involvement in the establishment of physical therapy goals: Effects on treatment outcome and quality of care. Advances in Physiotherapy 6:50–69.

Baker SM, Marshak HH, Rice GT, & Zimmerman GJ (2001). Patient participation in physical therapy goal setting. Physical Therapy 81(5):1118–1126.

Bassett SF & Petrie KJ (1999). The effect of treatment goals on patient compliance with physiotherapy exercise programmes. Physiotherapy 85(3):130–137.

Bell RA, Kravitz RL, Thom D, Krupat E, & Azari R (2002). Unmet expectations for care and the patient-physician relationship. Journal of General Internal Medicine 17(11):817–824.

Binder EF, Brown M, Sinacore DR, Steger-May K, Yarasheski KE, & Schechtman KB (2004). Effects of extended outpatient rehabilitation after hip fracture: A randomized controlled trial. JAMA 292:837–846.

Bradley EH, Bogardus ST, van Doorn C, Williams CS, Cherlin E, & Inouye SK (2000). Goals in geriatric assessment: Are we measuring the right outcomes? The Gerontologist 40(2):191–196.

Campbell R, Quilty B, & Dieppe P (2003). Discrepancies between patients' assessments of outcome: Qualitative study nested within a randomized controlled trial. British Medical Journal 326 252–253.

Cook C, Stickley L, Ramey K, & Knotts VJ (2005). Variables associated with occupational and physical therapy stroke rehabilitation utilization and outcomes. Journal of Allied Health 34(1):3–10.

Friedrich M, Gittler G, Halberstadt Y, Cermak T, & Heiller I (1998). Combined exercise and motivation program: Effect on the compliance and level of disability of patients with chronic low back pain: A randomized controlled trial. Archives of Physical Medicine and Rehabilitation 79:475–487.

Grimmer K, Sheppard L, Pitt M, Magarey M, & Trott P (1999). Differences in stakeholder expectations in the outcome of physiotherapy management of acute low back pain. International Journal for Quality in Health Care 11(2):155–162.

Indredavik B, Bakke F, Slordahl SA, Rokseth R, &

Haheim LL (1998). Stroke unit treatment improves long-term quality of life: A randomized controlled trial. Stroke 29(5):895–899.

Jette AM. (1995). Outcomes research: Shifting the dominant research paradigm in physical therapy. Physical Therapy 75:965–970.

Jette DU, Warren RL, & Wirtalla C (2005). The relation between therapy intensity and outcomes of rehabilitation in skilled nursing facilities. Archives of Physical Medicine and Rehabilitation 86(3):373–379.

Jia H, Uphold CR, Wu S, Chen GJ, & Duncan PW (2005). Predictors of changes in health-related quality of life among men with HIV infection in the HAART era. AIDS Patient Care STDS 19(6): 395–405.

Johnston MV & Granger CV. (1994). Outcomes research in medical rehabilitation: A primer and introduction to a series. American Journal of Physical Medicine and Rehabilitation 73(4): 296–303.

Kaplan SH, Greenfield S, & Ware JE. (1989). Assessing the effects of physician-patient interactions on the outcomes of chronic disease. Medical Care 27(3):S110–S127.

Lynn J & DeGrazia D (1991). An outcomes model of medical decision making. Theoretical Medicine 12:325–343.

Randall KE & McEwen IR (2000). Writing patient-centered functional goals. Physical Therapy 80(12):1197–1203.

Rothstein JM, Echternach JL, & Riddle DL (2003). The Hypothesis Oriented Algorithm for Clinicians II (HOAC II): A guide for patient management. Physical Therapy 83:455–470.

Starfield B, Wray C, Hess K, Gross R, Birk PS, & D'Lugoff BC (1981). The influence of patient-practitioner agreement on outcome of care. American Journal of Public Health 71(2): 127–131.

Tabor's Cyclopedic Medical Dictionary (2005). FA Davis Company, Philadelphia.

Tichenor CJ & Davidson JM (1997). Postprofessional clinical residency education. In KF Shepard & GM Jensen (eds.). Handbook of Teaching for Physical Therapists (pp 199–224). Boston, Butterworth-Heinemann.

Wennberg JE & Gittelsohn A (1982). Variations in medical care among small areas. Scientific American 246:120–134.

APPENDIX

Sample Portion of a Traditional Initial Evaluation Format

Patient Name: _____ Patient ID #: _____

Date of Birth/Age: _____ Date of Injury: ___ /___ / ___ Date of Surgery: ___ /___ /___

ICD-9 Code(s): _____ Diagnosis: _____

Referring Physician: _____ Referring Physician ID #: _____

Therapy Office (Site/Location): _____ Discipline: PT / OT

OBJECTIVE FINDINGS   Involved Region: Left / Right / N/A

Strength (0-5)   **Range of Motion**

Motion	Grade	Motion	PROM	AROM

How/Where Injury Occurred: Work Related?   Yes   No

Pertinent History:

Pain: Pain Scale: /10   Nature: constant / intermittent / localized / radiating

Functional Deficits / Additional Information:

Specific Treatment Plan:

Treatment Goals:

Projected Frequency / Duration of Treatment: Visits Requested:

Therapist Signature: Printed Therapist Name and License #:

The location for recording patient goals on this traditional form follows the examination findings.

Sample of an Outcome-Oriented Documentation Format

DEPARTMENT OF HEALTH AND HUMAN SERVICES
CENTERS FOR MEDICARE & MEDICAID SERVICES

PLAN OF TREATMENT FOR OUTPATIENT REHABILITATION

1. PATIENT'S LAST NAME	FIRST NAME	M.I.	2. PROVIDER NO.	3. HICN

4. PROVIDER NAME	5. MEDICAL RECORD NO. *(Optional)*	6. ONSET DATE	7. SOC. DATE

8. TYPE ☐ PT ☐ OT ☐ SLP ☐ CR ☐ RT ☐ PS ☐ SN ☐ SW	9. PRIMARY DIAGNOSIS *(Pertinent Medical D.X.)*	10. TREATMENT DIAGNOSIS	11. VISITS FROM SOC.

12. PLAN OF TREATMENT FUNCTIONAL GOALS	PLAN
GOALS *(Short Term)* ◄————————————	
OUTCOME *(Long Term)*	

13. SIGNATURE *(professional establishing POC including prof. designation)*	14. FREQ/DURATION *(e.g., 3/Wk. x 4 wk.)*

I CERTIFY THE NEED FOR THESE SERVICES FURNISHED UNDER THIS PLAN OF TREATMENT AND WHILE UNDER MY CARE ☐ N/A	17. CERTIFICATION
15. PHYSICIAN SIGNATURE ‖ 16. DATE	FROM ‖ THROUGH ‖ N/A
	18. ON FILE *(Print/type physician's name)* ☐

20. INITIAL ASSESSMENT *(History, medical complications, level of function at start of care. Reason for referral.)*	19. PRIOR HOSPITALIZATION
	FROM ‖ TO ‖ N/A

21. FUNCTIONAL LEVEL *(End of billing period)* PROGRESS REPORT ☐ CONTINUE SERVICES **OR** ☐ DC SERVICES

22. SERVICE DATES
FROM ‖ THROUGH

Form CMS-700-(11-91)

The location for recording patient goals on the CMS-700 form precedes the examination findings, a format more in keeping with an outcome approach to patient management.

EXERCISES

➤➤ Worksheet 2.1 Documentation Analysis

Use the following documentation analysis to determine how easily daily documentation processes will support collection of data for outcome studies. Use a blank initial evaluation form from the clinic. Circle the responses to the right that best reflect actual documentation practices. Compare the total to the scoring interpretation that follows.

Circle the appropriate score	Yes	No
I. DATA FORMATS		
Notes are in narrative form.	0	1
If yes, are there required headings?	1	0
Codes are printed on the forms to select.	3	0
Are codes entered by therapists?	1	0
If yes, do YOU ALWAYS fill them in?	2	1=usually 0=mostly no
Are therapists allowed to use their own abbreviations or measurement formats?	0=always	1=some 2=never
The PTs have agreed on how to document selected impairments and functions.	2	0
Documentation of selected impairments and functions is checked for compliance with the agreed upon standards.	3	0
II. DOCUMENT FORMATS		
Paper	0	NA
Electronic	3	NA
IIIA. ACCESS TO CHARTS		
Manual chart find and retrieval	0	NA
Computerized find, manual retrieval	1	0
Computerized find and retrieval	2	0
IIIB. ACCESS TO PATIENT DATA		
Paper system	0	NA
Spreadsheet list	1	
Database	3	NA
The database is searchable by patient diagnosis and can generate a list of patients I have treated.	2	0
I have searched the database by patient diagnosis and generated a list of patients I have treated.	3	

continued on page 39

Circle the appropriate score	Yes	No
IV. DOCUMENTATION REVIEW	2	0
We have an ongoing QA/CQI process that reviews patient documentation.		
V. DATA GENERATION	3	0
I have created a data set using my patient records.		
Total Score (Add all points)		

▶▶ Worksheet 2.2 Documentation Analysis Scoring Interpretation

Use the following score ranges to interpret how easily a documentation system will support data collection for outcome studies. Do not be dismayed if the score is low; there are more opportunities for improvement!

Section	Not ready for outcome studies	Potential to start simple outcome studies with some minor changes.	Solid foundation for starting outcome studies.
I. DATA FORMATS	0-4	5-7	8-14
II. DOCUMENT FORMATS	0	3	
III. ACCESS TO DATA	0	1-6	7-11
IV. DOCUMENT REVIEW	0	2	
V. DATA GENERATION	0	0	3
Total Score	0-9	10-17	18-31

Common Outcomes in Rehabilitation

KEY TERMS

Patient outcomes

Impairment outcomes

Functional outcomes

Provider outcomes

Service outcomes

Quality of life

Health-related

quality of life

Medical effectiveness

Patient satisfaction

Service satisfaction

Technical satisfaction

Humaneness satisfaction

Goods satisfaction

Access satisfaction

Atmospherics

Mortality

Morbidity

Cost-effectiveness

Cost-benefit

Cost-utility

Unit cost

Normative standard

Relative standard

Criterion reference

QALY

Q-TWiST

CHAPTER OUTCOMES

➤ Describe common domains of physical therapy outcomes.

➤ Describe outcomes found in other health-care literature.

There are many types of health service outcomes that can be measured. This chapter introduces the more common domains of outcomes that physical therapists find useful as well as examples of how they might be measured. It introduces several outcomes that have not been typically measured by physical therapy practices but for which there is increasing interest. Several medical outcome measures are described that are frequently reported in the literature and that physical therapists may find helpful to understand. This chapter does not describe specific measurement tools or instruments that can be used to generate data for outcome studies, except as examples to illustrate an approach to data collection or as an example from the literature. Because all outcome studies are relative to the questions that are asked and the environments that generate the data, specific measurement tools need to be examined on a case-by-case basis.

COMMON OUTCOME MEASURES IN REHABILITATION

Rehabilitation outcomes can be organized into three categories: patient outcomes, provider outcomes, and service outcomes. Each has its own perspective and uses outcome data for different purposes.

Physical therapy **patient outcomes** are those changes in the consequences of illness or injury that occur as a result of intervention. Examples of physical therapy patient outcomes include changes in function, social roles, rate of symptom recurrence, and occurrence of complications. Patient outcomes are usually observed or measured by physical therapists during clinical visits or follow-up contacts but are also reported by the patient. The reference point for patient outcomes is the patient; that is, patients will find these measures meaningful.

Provider outcomes are the result of service delivery activities, whether the provider is an individual or a group of clinicians. Provider outcomes include items that can be measured about clinicians, such as service consistency, intervention effectiveness, percentage of satisfied patients on caseload, service cost per provider, provider satisfaction, and knowledge. Impairment changes are also provider outcomes because they are indicators of intervention effectiveness that are meaningful to the clinician and typically have limited relevance to the patient. The reference point for provider outcomes in physical therapy is the physical therapist.

Service outcomes relate to the delivery of services within an institution, among similar institutions or across larger health-care systems. The reference point for service outcomes might be the administrators of a physical therapy practice or group of practices, an accreditation or management group that oversees the quality of care in an institution or type of health-care system, or government agencies that purchase services. Examples of service outcomes include overall patient satisfaction, utilization of procedures, variability in care, service costs and profits per diagnosis, staff retention and access, reimbursement patterns, referral rates, accreditation status, and comparisons of similar variables with other types of health-care systems. Service outcomes are often the basis for benchmarking processes, in which two or more similar facilities compare themselves on the same service outcome. There are many more audiences interested in service outcomes, so there is no single reference point.

This chapter will describe categories of outcomes that are found in the literature and provide examples of studies that use those outcomes.

PATIENT OUTCOMES

The following sections describe patient outcomes and approaches to measurement. In keeping with an outcome perspective to patient care, functional outcomes are the priority for patients. Changes in impairments are addressed in the section on Provider Outcomes, as impairment changes are indicators for the clinician (a means to an end) and not meaningful for patients.

Functional Outcomes

Functional outcomes are measures of the patient's ability to perform the tasks of everyday living. They include activities of daily living (ADL), instrumental activities of daily living (IADL), home and work activities, and goal-directed mobility skills. ADL refer to basic self-care tasks such as dressing, eating, bathing, and using the toilet. IADL refer to more complex tasks necessary for independent living, such as the ability to launder and fold clothes, prepare and clean-up from meals, and clean and maintain a home. Work-related tasks are the activities performed by patients where they are employed or volunteer their skills, such as lifting objects, filing, sitting at a computer to type, using telephones, or standing to use a cash register. Goal-directed mobility skills are skills needed to move within and between the environments in which the patient must function, such as within the home, from home to transportation, from transportation to work, and to and within medical, community, and vocational sites. As patients and environments can vary tremendously, functional outcomes are often specific to the individual patient's life roles and work settings.

Physical therapists are experts at identifying functional losses and designing intervention strategies to restore function, but *objective documentation* of changes in function has lagged behind documentation of impairments. Ideally, standardized measures would be used across settings for similar patients so that comparisons of patient outcomes would be based on common definitions and measures. Valid and reliable tools that standardize measurement of function have not been as readily available as those for measuring impairments. There is also a strong tradition in physical therapy of "creating our own" functional assessment or task evaluation tool. "Home-grown" tools are not always subjected to validity and reliability studies; however, they may be all that are available and serve to standardize documentation within a clinical practice.

Even when a valid and reliable tool is available, there are reasons it may not be used. The tool may not have been tested on similar patients, so there are concerns about its applicability. It may not fit easily into a clinic's documentation system, either because of physical size or the organization of medical records. The time to complete a standardized tool may be perceived as a burden, if time with a patient is limited. In some cases, a tool may ask for information that the clinician does not believe is necessary for a given patient or diagnosis; consequently, sections of the tool may be incomplete or not used at all. While there are many reasons why standardized measures or tools are not used regularly, they are the basis of systematic documentation, which

> ➤ *Many clinicians struggle with the role of pain as an impairment that is meaningful to patients. This author contends that although pain is an impairment that can be measured with reliability, most patients are more interested in being able to* function *with less pain than in the reduction of pain itself. Pain as an outcome measure is thus more relevant to the provider as an indicator of pain reduction techniques rather than as a patient outcome.*

is an essential component of outcome measurement. In the absence of a standardized tool, the clinician still has options for standardizing patient measures over time.

Option 1: Normative Standards

There are several standards against which function can be measured. One option is to measure against the gold standard of normal independent performance. In this case, the patient, regardless of diagnosis, is compared with a healthy, age-matched cohort, and their ability to perform functional activities is gauged. Comparison against age-matched, typically developing people naturally incorporates developmental readiness as well as the changes in speed or accuracy related to the physiology of normal development and aging. The benefit of comparing patients with age norms is that the norms often reflect the type of tasks that are relevant to that stage of life.

There is a limitation to comparing patients who have chronic conditions with age norms. The patients may need to readjust their expectations of function based on their diagnoses, such that chronological norms are not as relevant as diagnosis-related outcomes. Diagnosis-specific measurement tools will address those issues and activities that are typically difficult for a patient because of the diagnostic presentation. Diagnosis-related outcomes are continually changing as the profession explores more efficient interventions. One example of a changing functional outcome is evident in the literature on body weight–supported treadmill training (BSWTT). For decades, therapists did not expect to see significant changes in ambulation independence in patients with strokes beyond what they had achieved during the first 6–8 months. Studies using BSWTT with patients whose strokes occurred even 2 or more years previously are demonstrating significant changes in independent ambulation with relatively short, intense training periods (Hesse, et al., 2001). Thus, the norm for functional recovery is improving as interventions improve.

Option 2: Relative Standards

A second option for measuring functional outcomes is to use patients as their own measure of success. In this approach, the clinician compares the patient's perception of what is acceptable or desirable with the patient's current status. Each patient has unique goals, and improvement is documented when the level of patient independence increases beyond that of the patient's initial measures. An example of this technique is goal attainment scaling (Palisano, 1993), in which patient-specific goals are established with five levels of performance, two representing improvement beyond the goal and two representing performance levels below the desired goal (Box 3.1). The benefit of developing unique patient goals and performance criteria is that the goals have greater contextual meaning for the patient, which might influence motivation, cooperation, and success. The limitation of using such individualized goals is that patients cannot be compared with each other on the *content* of the goals because the goals and/or the criteria for performance are unique for each patient; however, *frequencies* of the number and types of goals met by patients can be quantified.

BOX 3.1

Example of Goal Attainment Scaling of Functional Outcomes

When supported at the pelvis, the child will:
- −2 = Sit without arching her trunk for 10 seconds (initial level of goal attainment)
- −1 = Sit without using her hands for support for 30 seconds
- 0 = Sit and use both hands to play with a toy for 60 seconds
- +1 = Sit with her trunk erect and use both hands to play with a toy for 60 seconds
- +2 = Sit erect and rotate her trunk to either side to reach for a toy

From Palisano R. (1993). Validity of goal attainment scaling in infants with motor delays. Physical Therapy 73:651–660.

Option 3: The Criterion Reference

A third option is to compare patient performance against a criterion reference for each task. The tools may or may not be diagnosis-specific. If they are diagnosis-specific, then the options for grading the task will include measurement of accommodations that are typical to the diagnosis. For criterion reference tools, the patient's performance of an activity is compared with a task analysis of that activity. Measurement includes the number of task steps that the patient can perform, the time to complete the task, and the ability to perform under selected conditions. The Rivermead ADL Scale (Lincoln & Edmans, 1990) was designed for patients with strokes and is an example of a diagnosis-specific criterion referenced scale (Box 3.2). The School Functional Assessment (Box 3.3) is an example of a criterion reference scale that crosses diagnostic labels but is specific to the elementary school environment.

BOX 3.2

Items From the Rivermead ADL Scale

Self Care	**Score**
Drinking	____
Comb hair	____
Wash face/hands	____
Makeup or shave	____
Clean teeth	____
Eating	____

Scores: 1 = Independent with/without aids
           OV = needs verbal supervision
           O = Dependent

From Lincoln NB, Edmans JA (1990). A re-validation of the Rivermead ADL Scale for elderly patients with stroke. Age and Ageing 19:19–24.

BOX 3.3

Sample Items From the School Functional Assessment, Part III Activity Performance Physical Tasks, "Up/Down Stairs".

1. Moves up and down single step (e.g., curb).	1 2 3 4
2. Walks/moves up/down a short flight of stairs (4–5 steps).	1 2 3 4
3. Walks/moves down a flight of stairs (at least 12 steps).	1 2 3 4
4. Walks/moves up a flight of stairs (at least 12 steps).	1 2 3 4
5. Walks/moves up and down a flight of stairs (at least 12 steps) with regular speed.	1 2 3 4
6. Walks/moves up and down stairs at regular speed when carrying an object.	1 2 3 4
Up/Down Stairs Raw Score	

1 = Does not perform, 2 = Partial performance, 3 = Inconsistent performance, 4 = Consistent performance.
From the School Function Assessment© 1998, The Psychological Corporation, San Antonio, TX.

Considerations in Choosing a Measurement Approach

The choice of measurement depends on the medical prognosis, the type of measures the clinician needs, the patient's goals, and the existence of valid and reliable tools to use. The benefit of using a standardized tool is that it allows for comparison of results across multiple settings. Measuring patients against an individualized or home-grown set of criteria does not allow for easy comparison of similar patients from other settings, but it may have more contextual relevance for the individual patient.

When the same measurement tool is used across multiple settings, data can be pooled to create larger data sets. Larger data sets provide more detailed understanding of the impact that different patient characteristics have on patient outcomes. Larger data sets also increase confidence that results are not affected by statistical or design errors. For example, a large data set is managed by the Uniform Data System for Medical Rehabilitation (UDSMR), which contains scores from the Functional Independence Measure (FIM) used at acute and subacute rehabilitation sites. As of 2001, the UDSMR had over 1400 member facilities that had contributed more than 2.5 million patient records to its databases. Many studies have been performed on the data sets, investigating such topics as the predictive values of FIM scores (Franchignoni, et al.,1998), perceived dependence at 2 years post stroke (Grimby, et al., 1998), and the usefulness of the total FIM score in patients with first strokes (Ring, et al.,1997). Another large data set is Focus on Therapeutic Outcomes, Inc. (FOTO), for outpatient physical therapy settings, which has over 550 institutions annually contributing approximately 110,000 patient records to its data set. The FOTO data have been used to study health outcomes in patients with knee impairments (Jette & Jette, 1996) and spinal impairments (Jette & Jette, 1996), as well as to describe the range of interventions provided to patients with musculoskeletal injuries (Jette & Delitto, 1997). For both the UDSMR and FOTO approaches, the tools used have undergone validity and reliability testing, and the clinicians contributing patient data are required to demonstrate an acceptable level of intra- and intertester reliability prior to contributing data.

Some standardized tools are specific to the treatment setting, which allows comparison among people in a similar stage of recovery. The LORS-II was designed to measure changes in patients in hospital-based rehabilitation settings (Posavac & Carey, 1987). The School Functional Assessment was designed to measure functional ability of children in elementary school settings (Coster, et al., 1998).

Another useful distinction among functional scales is whether they measure skill acquisition or skill application (Evans, Small, & Ling, 1995). Those measuring skill acquisition are generally designed for the earlier stages of recovery, when the environment is predictable and unchanging. Scales that measure skill application are focused on the person in natural environments. In these settings, the patient must constantly assess changing conditions against his or her own ability to function. A study by Doty, et al. (1999) illustrates the difference between skill acquisition and application. Children with and without disabilities were tested on the ability to catch a ball with a therapist in a one-to-one session (a predictable setting) and during a game of toss with peers (a natural environment). The performance of children with disabilities was higher during the predictable one-to-one session than when playing with peers, demonstrating that measures of skill acquisition were higher than skill application.

In summary, there are multiple methods for measuring functional status. Measurements include scores on standardized evaluations, the qualities of a skill, the number of component tasks or steps that can be completed within a larger activity, and the frequency of repetitions possible before a performance decrement is observed. The following are examples of studies that have used functional outcomes.

Examples From the Literature

Case Study Research: Charles, Lavinder, and Gordon (2001) studied the effects of 2 weeks of constraint-induced therapy on 3 children with hemiplegic cerebral palsy. They used the Jebsen-Taylor Test of Hand Function, a nondiagnostic specific test consisting of seven timed functional hand activities such as page turning, picking up small objects, and stacking checkers.

Descriptive Research: Kirk-Sanchez and Roach (2001) used retrospective data from the FIM as collected by the UDSMR. They found a positive correlation between the total hours of inpatient physical and occupational therapy services received and the level of independent mobility achieved at discharge for patients with orthopedic diagnoses.

Comparative Research: Ketelaar, et al. (2001) used a randomized block design to compare the effects of two treatment approaches on children with cerebral palsy. They concluded that functional skill performance in daily situations was greater after the children received functionally oriented therapy as compared with therapy focused on normalization of movement as measured by the Pediatric Evaluation of Disability Inventory.

Social/Role Outcomes

Social or role outcomes reflect the changes in social opportunity and participation that a patient experiences as a result of injury or illness. These outcomes include work capacity, spousal and parental functions, and recreation and avocation activities. Most scales combine assessment of function and social or role activity to measure access to opportunities, success in those opportunities, and perceptions of patient satisfaction with the opportunities. The Oswestry Low Back Pain Questionnaire is an example of a diagnosis-specific tool that combines questions about personal care independence, walking and sitting status, and assessment of travel opportunities and social life limitations (Fairbank & Pynsent, 2000).

Most patients are as interested in maintaining their social and mental health as they are in their physical health (Sherbourne, et al., 1999). The benefit of using a measure of social limitation is that it provides a reflection of the ultimate outcomes in patient care; that is, the return to prior levels of lifestyles. The challenge of interpreting these measures is that many life factors can affect the perception of satisfaction with role status. Changes in financial status, social support, and environmental access may all affect perceptions of health and role success (Aharony & Strasser, 1992; de Haan, et al., 1993). Teasing out the impact of physical therapy interventions thus becomes more difficult.

Two specific measurement concepts, quality of life and health-related quality of life, evaluate the patient's perceptions of overall life quality. These measures are appearing in physical therapy literature with increasing frequency.

Quality of Life Outcomes

Quality of life (QOL) can be defined in many ways, depending on the perspective of the evaluator. In its most basic definition, QOL refers to a person's assessment of satisfaction with life. If a group of people were asked, "How would you assess the quality of your life?" the responses might vary widely as well as be difficult to compare. In this broad question, QOL could refer to perceptions about health status, but it could also refer to perceptions of satisfaction with work, social life, community comfort, academic success, and financial status (de Haan, et al., 1993). It is easy to see that by repeating the question with each of those topics inserted (How would you assess the quality of your work life? your social life? your academic life?), responses might change.

In order to measure changes in QOL, a number of constructs have been developed to focus the interest of the evaluator. There is general consensus in the literature that any construct of QOL assesses multiple dimensions including the social, psychological, physical health, and functional abilities of the person at one point in time (de Haan, et al., 1993; Hoffman, Rouse, & Brin, 1995; Jenkins, 1992; Kaplan, Feeny, & Revicki, 1993; Testa & Nackley, 1994). How these constructs are assessed and the units of measurement reflected in the final rating of QOL are what make each tool or approach unique.

Health-Related Quality of Life Outcomes

Health-related quality of life (HRQOL) is a multidimensional assessment of life satisfaction as it relates to the person's state of health and the societal expectations of people who do or do not have disabilities (Hoffman, Rouse, & Brin, 1995; Jenkins, 1992). It is the more commonly used QOL construct in rehabilitation studies because it links health status with loss of function, two areas that physical therapists address. As with measures of QOL, there is consensus that the physical, psychological, social, economic, and functional domains should be included in any HRQOL scale. Jenkins (1992) suggests that there cannot be a single measure of HRQOL that could be applied to all patient populations; the actual items needed to measure HRQOL will differ based on the diagnostic grouping, the age of the patients, and the cultural and social expectations.

Assessment scales of HRQOL can be divided into three types: general health profiles, disease-specific scales, and scale batteries. General health profiles, such as the Medical Outcomes Study Short Form 36 or 12 (SF-36 or SF-12) (Stewart, Hays, & Ware,1988) or the Dartmouth COOP Charts (Kinirons, Weston, & Rai, 1998), address many health issues and can be used on many patient populations. Disease-specific scales, such as the Frenchay Activities Index for Stroke (Post & de Witte, 2003) or the Minnesota Living with Heart Failure questionnaire (Oldridge, Perkins, & Hodes, 2002), have been derived for specific conditions. Scale batteries, such as the Karnofsky Performance Status Scale (de Haan, et al., 1993), measure specific domains such as functional activities or cognitive processing (Hoffman, Rouse, & Brin, 1995).

HRQOL data are collected in one of two ways: self-administration or interviewer administration of a survey. For self-administered scales, the patient completes a survey independent of the clinician's assistance or presence. Answers are usually recorded by circling answers or filling in bubbles on a scan form; however, computer touch screens are increasingly popular because of their ease of use for patients and the ability to directly download answers into a larger data set. Interviewer-administered surveys can be completed face-to-face with the patient or by telephone. When a clinician assists the patient, there is room for discussion about how to interpret questions. This option does not exist when the patient self-administers the tool.

Impairment and functional limitation data are often collected by physical therapists at each patient visit in order to evaluate progress. In contrast, HRQOL data are typically collected at the beginning and end of intervention services to demonstrate an overall change. Some studies measure patients at selected intervals following discharge to describe the long-term effects of intervention services. Long-term studies of HRQOL provide an understanding of the long-term effectiveness of interventions, the rate of symptom reoccurrence that might go undetected, and they provide information about the prognosis of similar patients.

Examples From the Literature

Case Study Research: Kaplan (2000) describes the changes, using the SF-36, of a young woman 3–5 years post pontine hemorrhage, before and after receiving several home-based physical therapy sessions. The results demonstrated that although HRQOL scores rose initially, the scores did not parallel the continual and significant improvements in both function and role participation.

Comparative Research: DiFabio, et al. (1997) compared patients with chronic progressive multiple sclerosis who received outpatient rehabilitation for 1 year with patients who were on a waiting list and did not receive services for that year. The treatment group improved in six areas of health status on the SF-36, whereas the wait-list group had no changes.

Camp, et al. (2000) compared the HRQOL of 29 patients with congestive obstructive pulmonary disease before and after pulmonary rehabilitation. They used the SF-36 and the Chronic Respiratory Disease Questionnaire as HRQOL measures. Significant improvements were seen on both.

PROVIDER OUTCOMES IN REHABILITATION

Provider outcomes describe the efficiency, effectiveness, and satisfaction of an individual or group of clinicians. Provider outcomes have not been a major focus in physical therapy literature; however, trends in practice increasingly require all health-care providers to examine and report on their efficiency and effectiveness. Examples of clinician outcomes include measures of role changes, treatment variability, physical therapist satisfaction, success rates with different procedures, the costs of achieving certain outcomes, and the relationship of the level of clinician experience with selected outcomes. The following section explores some of the more prevalent outcomes of interest to providers.

Impairment Outcomes

Impairment outcomes are measures of changes at the body or tissue level that may occur as a result of intervention. While impairments happen to the patient, impairments as outcomes are more important to the clinician than to the patient. With the exception of changes in pain, most patients will not relate improvements in status by reporting impairment changes; rather, they report on an activity or function that is easier to complete. Examples of impairments that clinicians measure on patients include pain perception, strength, range of motion, coordination, endurance, circulation, and wound healing. The study of impairments provides insight into the healing processes of a condition and the application and effectiveness of interventions that were used. In some cases, impairment studies allow clinicians to challenge routine applications of interventions or to lay the foundations of an explanation for why certain interventions seem to work. Clark, et al. (1999) provides an example of an impairment study that sought to explain the effectiveness of stretching hip flexors in order to gain more range in the hip extensors. The premise of the study is initially counterintuitive, but the authors' rationale for the study is based on observations from clinical practice (Box 3.4).

BOX 3.4

An Impairment Study

Clark, et al. (1999) examined the effect of two anterior hip stretching techniques on range of motion during a passive straight-leg raise. Using a randomized 3-group pretest-post-test design to collect data on 60 nondisabled subjects, the researchers concluded that sagittal plane hold-relax stretching of the anterior hip muscles was more effective than static prone positioning and that both were more effective than supine rest for increasing hip extensor flexibility.

Impairments are typically more often documented than functional limitations (Turner, et al., 1999). This may be due to the fact that even small changes in impairment measures serve as comfortable indicators to both physical therapists and patients that interventions may be working. Changes in numerical measures of respiration rate, heart rate, strength, or range of motion are easy to record and compare and thus become motivating factors for continuing with a plan of care. Clinicians maintain strong intuitive assumptions that minimizing impairments will directly affect improvements in function, but there is little literature to support such direct cause-and-effect relationships (Jette, 1995). For example, an increase of 10° in shoulder flexion may or may not be enough to affect the overhead reach in a person with adhesive capsulitis. Although it is likely that increasing shoulder flexion will eventually improve the patient's ability to reach overhead into cabinets or to brush her hair, functional independence may also change by the patient's being provided adaptive equipment or by therapy addressing weakness within the available range. Therefore, changes in function may not be a direct effect of increasing range of motion but rather by using a different intervention approach or by addressing a different impairment.

The tools for measuring impairments are usually specific to the impairment. Thus, a goniometer is used to measure range of motion; an isokinetic dynamometer is used to measure force; and a force plate can quantify pressure. During the past three decades, faster and more powerful computers and programs have allowed for greater accuracy or efficiency in measuring impairment characteristics. A manual goniometer permits measurement of a static joint, but it cannot be used to measure changes in joint angles during motion. An electrogoniometer, however, can be strapped onto the limb segments around a joint and can measure both static and moving joint angles and communicate the degrees of movement to a computer. These two-dimensional raw data can then be viewed, plotted, and analyzed mathematically. A computerized motion analysis laboratory uses even more sophisticated methods for collecting data on joint angles. Infrared sensors, light-emitting diodes, and video cameras collect data on joint angles and provide three-dimensional information on joint angle changes. Thus, technology has provided three ways to measure joint angles with increasing detail, accuracy, and speed, and each technique serves a different purpose. When choosing a measurement tool to study impairments, it is important to determine the type of data that *needs* to be collected rather than be guided by the type of data that *can* be collected because the technology is available.

It is important to establish the reliability of an instrument for its ability to measure impairments. It is not enough to accept the information provided by an equipment designer or vendor as to the reliability of the tool. Therapists need to establish their own reliability when using the tool in practice. Berry, et al. (1999) demonstrated that even though a tool may be considered reliable, the level of reliability may differ based on the experience of the individual therapist (Box 3.5).

Examples From the Literature

Case Study Research: Kirsch and Myslinski (1999) documented pre- and postintervention measures on five aerobic conditioning variables in their case reports of 2 people with multiple sclerosis who participated in a 3-month fitness and education program. These variables were: resting heart rate and

---

BOX 3.5

Example of an Instrument Reliability Study

Berry, et al. (1999) tested the reliability of the KT-1000 arthrometer and found that experienced physical therapists had greater inter-rater and intertrial reliability than novice physical therapists. Although the sample of therapists is small, the data provide support for the need to train therapists in the use of the instrument.

---

blood pressure, workload maximum, metabolic equivalents, and VO_2 maximum.

Descriptive Research: Lehman and McGill (2001) describe the amount of electromyographic activity in different regions of the abdominal musculature during a variety of typical abdominal exercises.

Comparative Research: Ginn, et al. (1997) used a randomized controlled clinical trial to study the efficacy of physical therapy treatment for shoulder pain as measured by pain ratings, range of motion, and abduction force.

Clinician Role Development

The roles of physical therapists are continually evolving, from the start as a student and onward as the profession changes in practice. There is a growing body of literature that reflects the study of how professional skills are acquired and of how roles change. Teschendorf and Nemshick (2001) describe faculty perceptions of how they influence student professional socialization. Lopopolo (2001) developed the Professional Role Behaviors Survey to describe the roles of physical therapists among different organizational structures. Understanding how roles change as practice environments change or as practice acts change can provide important data to support curricular changes, continuing education, and organizational structures.

Clinician/Physical Therapist Satisfaction

Clinician satisfaction is a measure of work satisfaction. This construct is important to managers who hope to develop and retain staff, improve productivity, reduce absenteeism, and attract new staff as growth occurs (Akroyd, et al., 1994). Work satisfaction consists of two main clusters of variables: intrinsic variables, which are tasks that are completed, and extrinsic variables, which relate to the social and organizational environment. Some of the variables that contribute to work satisfaction include the level of interest in and reward from work-related tasks, autonomy in decision making, working conditions, salary, relationship with colleagues, relationship with supervisors, and overall satisfaction with work (Akroyd, et al., 1994). Studies of clinician satisfaction are more prevalent in the nursing literature, but studies of physical therapists (Schwertner, et al., 1987), physical therapy faculty (Harrison & Kelly, 1996), physical therapist assistants (Ellis, Connell, &

Ellis-Hill, 1998) are available to provide some indication of the factors that may affect role satisfaction.

Examples From the Literature

Descriptive Research: Akroyd, et al. (1994) surveyed physical and occupational therapists to determine which intrinsic and extrinsic variables were significant predictors of satisfaction in two settings. Regression analysis identified that "involvement" and "general work conditions" were the strongest predictors of work satisfaction in ambulatory care centers and hospital settings.

SERVICE OUTCOMES

Service outcomes are related to the management and administration of health service delivery and look at the overall effect of providing services to patients. Examples of service outcomes include patient satisfaction, service costs and profits, reimbursement or denial rates, and staff retention. This section will explore two of the more common service outcome measures.

Patient Satisfaction

Patient satisfaction is one of the most common service outcome measures. Despite its prevalence, "patient satisfaction" is a difficult term to define because it depends on the perspective of the interested party and because there are many facets of health-care delivery that can be measured (Avis, Bond, & Arthur, 1995; Hutton & Richardson, 1995; Leiter, et al., 1994). There is widespread acceptance of the concept of patient satisfaction by patients and service providers, but it is rare to find agreement on the definition of the concept (Rees Lewis, 1994) or evidence of its impact on the delivery of services (Aharony & Strasser,1992). At the most basic level, patient satisfaction relates to patients' *perceptions* of the care they receive.

The measurement of patient satisfaction is based on assumptions that patients have expectations of health care, that the expectations can be judged according to some qualitative criteria, and that the judgments result in some level of satisfaction or dissatisfaction. The problem with these assumptions is that studies suggest that patients may not have expectations of care until after the care is rendered or that expectations are not based on what they think will or should happen but rather on what would or should not happen (Avis, Bond, & Arthur, 1995). Additionally, it is not clear *which* aspects of care are related to patient expectations (Avis, Bond, & Arthur, 1995). Even if expectations exist, it is not clear whether judgments about satisfaction are related to patient expectations or to other variables, such as perceptions of health status, perceptions of caregiver competence, sociodemographic variables, age, gender, or patients' own perceived roles as patients (Avis, Bond, & Arthur, 1995; Keith, 1998). It is also not known if the items chosen for measurement of satisfaction by the service providers are related in any way to patient expectations; assessment of patient satisfaction may really reflect items that patients care little about (Avis, Bond, & Arthur, 1995).

There are some methodological challenges to measuring patient satisfaction. Patients may be reluctant to disclose satisfaction if they think their opinion might influence future services, or they may not complete the surveys because of cognitive deficits, thus biasing the respondent pool (Keith, 1998; Roush & Sonstroem, 1999). The timing of the survey completion, the balance of positive and negative service descriptors, the use of incentives with a survey (such as including a pen or receiving a gift for completion), the use of a proxy who completes the form for the patient, and the patient's age can affect the response rate and the resulting levels of satisfaction (Aharony & Strasser,1992; Avis, Bond, & Arthur,1995; Seibert, et al., 1999).

Despite a lack of consensus about how to measure patient satisfaction, service quality and consumer satisfaction are important concepts for marketing health-care services, and attempts to measure them are on the increase (Gerszten, 1998). Studies have shown that satisfaction is related to patient behavior, such as continued use of medical services, maintained use of a specific provider, and compliance with care (Aharony & Strasser, 1992; Bell, et al., 2002; Keith, 1998;). Conversely, patients with unmet expectations tend to be less satisfied and subsequently use more health services (Bell, et al., 2002). As satisfaction is correlated with improved patient compliance (Keith, 1998), and improved compliance is assumed to improve intervention outcomes, patient satisfaction continues to be an important concept to measure.

In keeping with a growing trend to understanding patient satisfaction with physical therapy services, the American Physical Therapy Association published a compendium of patient satisfaction tools in 1995. These tools were contributed voluntarily by clinics in response to a request to the membership to share the instruments they use. The variety of settings and formats of the surveys submitted support the point that clinics are interested in patient satisfaction; however, none of the forms had been subjected to psychometric testing to determine content validity or reliability. In response to growing interest in patient satisfaction, a variety of tools have been developed and have been subjected to validity and reliability testing in clinical settings (Beattie, et al., 2005; Goldstein, Elliott, & Guccione, 2000; Roush, et al., 1999; Seibert, 1999). Because patient satisfaction is recognized to be a multidimensional construct, most surveys include questions about multiple constructs. The following sections describe the types of constructs that are often measured in patient satisfaction surveys.

Service Satisfaction

This is satisfaction with the act of interacting with a service provider. It cannot be separated from the place where it occurs or the person who provides the service. The perception of satisfaction is highly variable, depending on the expectations of the consumer. Additionally, the focus is on the process of service delivery, not just on a single outcome of service (Hutton & Richardson, 1995).

Technical or Competence Satisfaction

This satisfaction concerns the patient's perception that the provider is knowledgeable about the patient's condition and is able to perform the necessary examination, evaluation, and treatment procedures in a comfortable and efficient way (Goldstein, Elliott, & Guccione, 2000). It is a type of service satisfaction.

Humaneness Satisfaction

This is the patient's perception of the provider's "warmth," caring, willingness to listen, appropriateness of nonverbal and verbal behaviors, and respect for the patient (Rees Lewis, 1994).

Goods Satisfaction

This is satisfaction with a product or item that can be used regardless of where it is produced. It is easier to assess satisfaction with goods than with services because patients' expectations of goods are more consistent over time and are very focused on what the goods are meant to do. In contrast, expectations of service can change with each encounter according to patients' perceptions of their own change (or lack of change) in status (Hutton & Richardson, 1995).

Atmospherics

This is the environment in which services are delivered. Designing the environment to match the targeted consumers has long been valued in the retail world and in private practice settings; however, measurement of the influence of the environment on patient satisfaction with service delivery is still in its early stages. Issues such as office organization, crowding, perceptions of how an office is supposed to look, and how expensive the furnishings look relative to the clientele served influence patients as to whether they want to return for services and whether they would recommend the clinician's services to others (Hutton & Richardson, 1995).

Access Satisfaction

This satisfaction results from the convenience with which services are scheduled, the hours of service, the distance to service, and perceived availability (Rees Lewis, 1994). This includes the ease with which a person can physically access services; for example, the ease of parking or proximity to public transportation, signs to find the clinic, ease of entrance and egress, and the ease of access to elevators. It can also include access to the clinician by telephone or through flexible scheduling.

Examples From the Literature

Descriptive Research: Elliot-Burke and Pothast (1997) identify the top five service issues contributing to overall patient satisfaction in outpatient orthopedic rehabilitation settings. They include receiving an explanation of treatment, personalized attention, number of different treating clinicians, how informed the clinician is of the patient's case, and the amount of patient input into setting treatment goals. Seibert, et al. (1999) demonstrate that different types of patient services and locations are related to different dimensions of patient expectations and levels of satisfaction.

Cost Outcomes

Cost accounting and valuation of services are probably the fastest growing approaches to measuring physical therapy outcomes. Two trends have accelerated the interest in cost-effectiveness outcomes. First, the federal government's interest in health-care access and allocation of financial resources has forced all levels of the health-care industry to focus on improving national access and effectiveness. The second change occurred in the health insurance industry as business management shifted from indemnity plans to managed care plans. In the former, health risk, financial risk, and the effectiveness of new treatments were reviewed for claims purposes; in the latter, management of medical care was used to control or reduce risk, with the assumption that reduced risk would reduce the costs of care. Thus, the need to assign costs, to determine outcomes, and to compare the value of services relative to costs has become part of the process of business management (Stewart, 1993). Now, as many physical therapy services are being provided both directly and indirectly by managed care organizations, physical therapists are being asked to produce cost-related outcomes as well.

There are many categories of costs that need to be accounted for when determining the full cost of services. These include expenses related to operating costs, depreciation of capital expenses (e.g., equipment, buildings), and the value of donated goods and services (e.g., volunteers or student clinicians, vehicles, office equipment). Direct and indirect costs are two categories of operating costs. Unfortunately, there is little consensus as to which items fall into each category.

Direct costs are most often identified as the tangible costs associated with the provision of service, such as the cost of disposables, patient equipment, and provider time in wages and benefits. Some consider facility expenses as a type of direct cost, whereas others consider it a type of indirect cost (Luce & Simpson, 1995).

Indirect costs come from expenses that do not have a transfer of money but for which there is a financial consequence (Whetten-Goldstein, et al., 2000) or that have multiple purposes or that are spread across many patients (Luce & Simpson,1995). Indirect costs that are spread across patients include facility rent and utility costs, equipment costs, administrator salaries, and marketing costs. Indirect costs that are not associated with an observable transfer of money include the cost of lost earnings through lost workdays or missed promotions and the cost of informal care provided by family members (Luce & Simpson, 1995; Whetten-Goldstein, et al., 2000). Intangible costs include the pain and suffering that a patient and family endure because of a disability (Whetten-Goldstein, et al., 2000).

The following are descriptions of cost-related measures in the literature. These terms do not have standardized, mutually exclusive definitions associated with them. They can have an array of operational definitions, depending on the perspective of who is writing about them. The following list is presented only to provide familiarity with the terms and some of their more common uses.

Unit Cost

This is the cost to produce or deliver one unit of a product or service and incorporates both direct and indirect costs of production. Units of service differ, depending on the provider and setting. For rehabilitation services, one unit may refer to a single treatment, a single period spent with a patient, or a single patient-day. In outpatient settings, the unit is based on time, with 15-minute increments being most common. In home-care settings, the unit cost may be defined per treatment (Hagen, 1999). Unit cost can also refer to the cost of a product, such as an orthotic or piece of durable equipment.

Cost-Effectiveness

This is a comparison of the cost to produce the same outcome by similar providers or service delivery systems. The provider or system that costs the least to achieve the same outcome is considered the most cost-effective. This outcome measure does not factor in the quality of service or any results of having provided the service. Later uses of the term describe a broader decision-making process that accounts for benefits measured in terms of natural health units, such as the life-years gained as a result of service or intervention (Luce & Simpson, 1995). Examples of provider cost-effectiveness includes the costs of achieving specific patient outcomes by novice and master clinicians and the costs of providing the service in an office versus a home setting.

Cost-Benefit

This is the positive benefit of providing services relative to the cost or negative aspects of providing the service (Block, 2006). When used in medical care studies, the most traditional measure of benefit has been in the monetary units (dollars) needed to produce added life-years (Luce & Simpson, 1995). Medication comparisons are the most familiar cost-benefit studies, where the cost of a generic form of a medication is compared with the cost of the brand-name form. Cost-benefit measures are appropriate for the goals of *medical intervention* because an immediate effect is often observable following an intervention. Cost-benefit studies on *rehabilitation* are less prevalent because interventions are more variable, and patient outcomes are often measured differently among clinicians and clinical settings. Examples of rehabilitation cost-benefit outcomes include the results of delivering interventions immediately versus the results of delaying intervention and the affect on patient recovery; the costs related to improved functional independence versus the need for assistance; and the costs of facilitating return to work versus continued disability status for a company or for society.

Cost-Utility

This is an estimate of patient preferences for different health states relative to the length and quality of life and available interventions (Haas, 1993; Luce & Simpson, 1995). These health states range from normal and healthy through death. It is a relatively new approach, for which there are many debates about how to estimate preferences, but it may be a very useful concept for rehabilitation. Many patients cannot return to their premorbid level of functioning or quality of life. In addition, patients with chronic conditions may have a variety of alternative approaches for managing their conditions over time. Measuring the match between patient preferences for a particular level of function or health state and the level actually achieved by different interventions may yield meaningful outcome measures that assist with clinical decision making and long-range patient management. For example, Haas (1993) evaluated the cost-utility of physical therapy intervention for a variety of orthopedic conditions and determined that the value was good compared with other interventions. In contrast, van den Hout, et al. (2005) concluded that usual care had better cost-utility than high-intensity exercise classes for people with rheumatoid arthritis.

Examples From the Literature

Cost-Effectiveness Research: In a retrospective study of 135 patients undergoing total hip arthroplasty, Gahimer, et al. (1996) demonstrated that preoperative patient education made no difference in patient outcomes, complication rates, levels of ambulation, or discharge to home. This type of study provides physical therapists with cost-effectiveness evidence that a well-accepted and well-intended intervention might increase the cost of service without improving outcomes.
Cost-Benefit Research: Freburger (2000) retrospectively examined the utilization of physical therapy services and its correlation with cost of care and discharge to home for patients who had a total hip arthroplasty. The cost-benefit results suggested that increased use of physical therapy was correlated with lower total cost of care and higher probability of discharge to home.
Cost-Benefit Research: Hamilton, et al. (1999) conducted a cross-sectional study on the cost of service for 109 patients with spinal cord injuries who had been treated at one of two regional medical centers. Inverse correlations were found between current total and component FIM scores and the minutes of assistance, cost of durable goods, and hours of paid help per day. That is, the lower FIM scores representing more severe limitations were correlated with higher costs of postrehabilitation care.

MEDICAL OUTCOMES

Medical outcomes have traditionally focused on several areas: morbidity and mortality rates, treatment effectiveness, and diagnostic accuracy. Medical sociologists have been more interested in such constructs as quality-adjusted life-years, which accounts for the quality of life gained as a result of intervention. Although the outcomes of medical intervention are important to physical therapists, they are not substitutes for rehabilitation outcomes. Descriptions of the following medical outcomes are provided because they are typically reported in medical and pharmaceutical outcome studies.

Morbidity and Mortality Rates

Morbidity refers to the ratio of sick to well in a community, or to the frequency of complications that follows a medical intervention. Morbidity rates are specific to diagnoses and related medical procedures. Despite a long history of morbidity rates, not all definitions of morbidity are consistent among studies of the same procedures. For example, in a study of four adverse surgical outcomes, variations in the definition of wound infection limited the ability to compare outcomes from different institutions (Bruce, et al., 2001). Other variables that affect the accuracy of morbidity rates include variations in the rating scales used to assess adverse results, duration of follow-up to determine adverse outcomes, and the validity of patient self-report about negative outcomes (Bruce, et al., 2001).

Mortality refers to the rate of death as a result of medical intervention. Although there is more consistency in the definition of mortality among institutions, the duration of follow-up time after discharge from a medical procedure varies (Bruce, et al., 2001). The challenge is to determine the amount of time after a medical procedure for which the cause of death is ascribed to that procedure. If mortality follow-up times vary greatly, then those studies with longer follow-up periods will more likely have higher mortality rates than those studies with immediate follow-ups.

These two rates are often reported when medical procedures are studied under controlled conditions as well as in epidemiological studies of a particular disease. They are the most often reported rates in medical outcome studies (Bailit, Federico, & McGivney, 1995).

Medical Treatment Effectiveness

Treatment effectiveness refers to the degree with which a medical intervention is able to cure a disease or condition. The absence of disease, the elimination of recurrence of a disease, and the comparative effectiveness of two treatments for the same condition are frequently reported medical outcomes. Medical treatment effectiveness differs from rehabilitation effectiveness in that rehabilitation services do not necessarily attempt to cure a condition. Rather, rehabilitation services seek to improve function, whether through recovery of lost skills or by teaching patients to accommodate safely to their conditions.

Quality-Adjusted Life-Years

Quality-adjusted life-years (QALY) is the assessment of duration of life weighed against the quality of that life (Ganiats, Miller, & Kaplan, 1995; Jenkins, 1992). QALY is prevalent in medical literature where there are two or more distinct strategies for treating a diagnosis that has a known lifespan estimate. QALY provides a comparison of one treatment over another to extend life expectancy relative to the quality of the life the person would have. The dilemma of the patient to be treated for cancer is a common example. Often, the choice must be made between a treatment that will extend life for several years but requires enduring uncomfortable treatments and side effects, or a less aggressive treatment that ensures greater physical comfort but without as much extension of time.

QALY is determined by measuring health-related quality of life in patients at specific intervals during a period that generally includes some form of intervention. Plotting the HRQOL scores against time produces a curve, under which is the estimate of QALY for a single patient. When the area under the curve is averaged for many patients, an average QALY for a sample or population can be determined (Ganiats, Miller, & Kaplan, 1995). QALYs can be compared when the interventions used for one sample of patients are different from another sample of patients. Ganiats, Miller, and Kaplan (1995) describe the strengths and limitations of determining QALY by this and several other methods. Although it is not a measure without bias, it is one that is commonly used in league tables that compare the outcomes of different treatment approaches for medical management of diseases, particularly terminal diseases. It is not a measure that has been applied to rehabilitation because the expected outcomes of care change to provision of support rather than recovery of function when a patient has limited survival expectancies.

Quality-Adjusted Time Without Symptoms and Toxicities

Q-TWiST is the acronym for quality-adjusted time without symptoms and toxicities. It is a quality-adjusted survival analysis in which the estimated survival time for a patient is adjusted according to the quality of life experienced (Schwartz, Cole, & Gelber, 1995). It has also been used primarily for patients with terminal diseases who have a choice between two or more strategies for medical management. More recently, its adaptation is being explored for use with patients with neurological diseases (Schwartz, Cole, & Gelber, 1995). For example, in a patient with cancer, the estimated survival time for the specific type and severity of cancer is adjusted according to the trade-offs of discomfort and chance of recurrence secondary to treatments of chemotherapy, radiation therapy, surgery, and any such combinations. Q-Twist provides a statistical means of comparing the benefits and side-effects of different interventions for the same diagnosis.

SUMMARY

This chapter describes a variety of patient and provider outcomes that can be measured. Outcome studies in physical therapy have typically centered on impairment outcomes. Changes in health service delivery expectations have increased the interest in measuring functional outcomes and have fostered more interest in other types of outcomes, such as patient satisfaction and cost analyses.

References

Aharony L & Strasser S (1992). Patient satisfaction: What we know about and what we still need to explore. Medical Care Review 50(1):49–79.

Akroyd D, Wilson S, Painter J, & Figuers C (1994). Intrinsic and extrinsic predictors of work satisfaction in ambulatory care and hospital settings. Journal of Allied Health 23:155–164.

Avis M, Bond M, & Arthur A (1995). Satisfying solutions? A review of some unresolved issues in the measurement of patient satisfaction. Journal of Advanced Nursing. 22:316–322.

Bailit H, Federico J, & McGivney W (1995). Use of outcomes studies by a managed care organization: Valuing measured treatment effects. Medical Care 33(4):AS216–AS225.

Beattie P, Turner C, Dowda M, Michener L, & Nelson R (2005). The MedRisk instrument for measuring patient satisfaction with physical therapy care: A psychometric analysis. Journal of Orthopaedic & Sports Physical Therapy. 35(1): 24–32.

Bell R, Kravitz RL, Thom D, Krupat E, & Azari R (2002). Unmet expectations for care and the patient-physician relationship. Journal of General Internal Medicine 17(11):817–24.

Berry J, Kramer K, Binkley J, Binkley GA, Stratford P, Hunter S, & Brown K (1999). Error estimates in novice and expert raters for the KT-1000 arthrometer. Journal of Orthopaedic and Sports Physical Therapy 29:49–55.

Block DJ (2006). Measuring cost effectiveness. In Healthcare Outcomes Management: Strategies for Planning and Evaluation. Jones and Bartlett Publishers, Sudbury, MA.

Bruce J, Russell EM, Mollison J, & Krukowski ZH (2001). The measurement and monitoring of surgical adverse events. Health Technology Assessment 5(22):1–194.

Camp PG, Appleton J, & Reid WD (2000). Quality of life after pulmonary rehabilitation: Assessing change using quantitative and qualitative methods. Physical Therapy 80:986–995.

Charles J, Lavinder G, & Gordon AM (2001). Effects of constraint-induced therapy on hand function in children with hemiplegic cerebral palsy. Pediatric Physical Therapy 13:68–76.

Clark S, Christiansen A, Hellman DF, Hugunin JW, & Hurst KM (1999). Effect of ipsilateral anterior thigh soft tissue stretching on passive unilateral straight-leg raise. Journal of Orthopedic and Sports Physical Therapy 29:4–12.

Coster WJ, Deeney T, Haltiwanger J, & Haley SM (1998). School Functional Assessment. The Psychological Corporation/Therapy Skill Builders, San Antonio, TX.

de Haan R, Aaronson N, Limburg M, Hewer RL, & van Crevel H (1993). Measuring quality of life in stroke. Stroke 24:320–327.

DiFabio RP, Choi T, Soderberg J, & Hansen CR (1997). Health-related quality of life for patients with progressive multiple sclerosis: Influence of rehabilitation. Physical Therapy 77(12): 1704–1716.

Doty AK, McEwen IR, Parker D, & Laskin J (1999). Effects of testing context on ball skill performance in 5-year-old children with and without developmental delay. Physical Therapy 79(9):818–826.

Ellis B, Connell NAD, & Ellis-Hill C (1998). Role, training and job satisfaction of physiotherapy assistants. Physiotherapy 84(12):608–16.

Evans RW, Small L, & Ling JS (1995). Independence in the home and community. In PK Landrum, ND Schmidt & A McLean, Jr. (eds.). Outcome oriented rehabilitation: Principles, strategies, and tools for effective program management (p 102). Gaithersburg, MD: Aspen Publishers.

Fairbank JCT & Pynsent PB (2000). The Oswestry Disability Index. Spine 25(22):2940–2953.

Franchignoni F, Tesio L, Martino MT, Benevolo E, & Castagna M. (1988). Length of stay of stroke rehabilitation inpatients: Prediction through the functional independence measure. Annali dell Istituto Speriore di Sanita. 34(4):463–467.

Freburger JK (2000). An analysis of the relationship between the utilization of physical therapy ser-vices and outcomes of care for patients after total hip arthroplasty. Physical Therapy 80(5):448–458.

Gahimer JE, Forsyth E, Domholdt E, Lewis MN, Corbin KE, & Rosier T (1996). A retrospective study on the effectiveness of preoperative patient education on postoperative outcomes and efficiency of care in patients undergoing total hip arthroplasty. Issues on Aging 19(1): 10–13.

Ganiats TG, Miller CJ, & Kaplan RM (1995). Comparing the quality-adjusted life-year output of two treatment arms in a randomized trial. Medical Care 33:AS245–AS254.

Gerszten PC. (1998). Outcomes research: A review. Neurosurgery Online 43:1145–1155.

Ginn KA, Herbert RD, Khouw W, & Lee R (1997). A randomized, controlled clinical trial of a treatment for shoulder pain. Physical Therapy 77(8):802–811.

Goldstein MS, Elliott SD, & Guccione AA (2000). The development of an instrument to measure satisfaction with physical therapy. Physical Therapy 80:853–863.

Grimby G, Andren E, Daving Y, & Wright B (1988). Dependence and perceived difficulty in daily activities in community-living stroke survivors 2 years after stroke: A study of instrumental structures. Stroke 29(9):1843–1849.

Haas M (1993). Evaluation of physiotherapy using cost-utility analysis. Australian Journal of Physiotherapy 39(3):211–216.

Hagen C (1999). The business of rehabilitation: Where does all the money go? In Rehabilitation in Managed Care: Controlling Cost, Ensuring Quality (pp. 28–29). Aspen Publishers, Gaithersburg, MD.

Hamilton BB, Deutsch A, Russell C, Fiedler RC, & Granger CV (1999). Relation of disability costs to function: Spinal cord injury. Archives of Physical Medicine and Rehabilitation 80:385–391.

Harrison AL & Kelly DG (1996). Career satisfaction of physical therapy faculty during their pretenure years. Physical Therapy 76(11):1202–1218.

Hesse S, Werner C, Bardeleben A, & Barbeau H (2001). Body weight-supported treadmill training after stroke. Current Atherosclerosis Reports 3(4):287–294.

Hoffman LG, Rouse MW, & Brin BN (1995). Quality of life: A review. Journal of the American Optometric Association 66:281–289.

Hutton JD & Richardson LD (1995).Healthscapes: The role of the facility and physical environment on consumer attitudes, satisfaction, quality assessments and behaviors. Health Care Management Review 20:48–61.

Jenkins DC (1992). Assessment of outcomes of health intervention. Social Science and Medicine 35:367–375.

Jette A (1995). Outcomes research: Shifting the dominant research paradigm in physical therapy. Physical Therapy 75:965–970.

Jette AM & Delitto A (1997). Physical therapy treatment choices for musculoskeletal impairments. Physical Therapy 77(2):145–154.

Jette DU & Jette AM (1996). Physical therapy and health outcomes in patients with knee impairments. Physical Therapy 76(11):1178–1187.

Jette DU & Jette AM (1996). Physical therapy and health outcomes in patients with spinal impairments. Physical Therapy 76(9):930–945.

Kaplan RM, Feeny D, & Revicki DA (1993). Methods for assessing relative importance in preference-based outcomes measures. Quality of Life Research 2:467–475.

Kaplan S (2000). Use of a quality of life measure with a young woman at three to five years post pontine hemorrhage: Case report. Neurology Report 24:152–158.

Keith RA (1998). Patient satisfaction and rehabilitation services. Archives of Physical Medicine and Rehabilitation 79:1122–1128.

Ketelaar M, Vermeer A, 't Hart H, van Petegem-van Beek E, & Helders PJM (2001). Effects of a functional therapy program on motor abilities of children with cerebral palsy. Physical Therapy 81(9):1534–1545.

Kinirons MT, Weston B, & Rai GS (1998). Use of COOP charts in the day hospital. Archives of Gerontology and Geriatrics 26:113–117.

Kirk-Sanchez NJ & Roach KE (2001). Relationship between duration of therapy services in a comprehensive rehabilitation program and mobility at discharge in patients with orthopedic problems. Physical Therapy 81:888–895.

Kirsch NR & Myslinski MJ (1999). The effect of a personally designed fitness program on the aerobic capacity and function of two individuals with multiple sclerosis. Physical Therapy Case Reports 2(1):19–26.

Lehman GJ & McGill SM (2001). Quantification of the differences in electromyographic activity magnitude between the upper and lower portion of the rectus abdominis muscle during selected trunk exercises. Physical Therapy 81:1096–1101.

Leiter P, Nettles C, Santopoalo R, & Velozo CA (1994). Outcomes research in outpatient orthopedics. Rehabilitation Management Aug-Sept:104–109.

Lincoln NB & Edmans JA (1990). A re-validation of the Rivermead ADL Scale for elderly patients with stroke. Age and Ageing 19:19–24.

Lopopolo RB (2001). Development of the Professional Role Behaviors Survey (PROBES). Physical Therapy 81(7):1317–1327.

Luce BR & Simpson K (1995). Methods of cost-effectiveness analysis: Areas of consensus and debate. Clinical Therapeutics 17:109–125.

Oldridge N, Perkins A, & Hodes Z (2002). Comparison of three heart disease–specific health-related quality of life instruments. Monaldi Archives for Chest Disease 58(1):10–18.

Palisano R (1993). Validity of goal attainment scaling in infants with motor delays. Physical Therapy 73:651–660.

Posavac EJ & Carey RG (1987). Using a level of function scale (LORS-II) to evaluate the success of inpatient rehabilitation programs. NLN Publications (21–2195):241–246.

Post MWM & de Witte LP (2003). Good inter-rater reliability of the Frenchay Activities Index in stroke patients. Clinical Rehabilitation 17(5):548–552.

Rees Lewis, J (1994). Patient views on quality care in general practice: Literature review. Social Science and Medicine 39:655–670.

Ring H, Feder M, Schwartz J, & Samuels G (1997). Functional measures of first-stroke rehabilitation inpatients: Usefulness of the Functional Independence Measure total score with a clinical rationale. Archives of physical Medicine and Rehabilitation 78(6):630–635.

Roush SE & Sonstroem RJ (1999). Development of the Physical Therapy Outpatient Satisfaction Survey (PTOPS). Physical Therapy 79:159–170.

Schwartz CE, Cole BF, & Gelber RD (1995). Measuring patient-centered outcomes in neurologic disease: Extending the Q-twist method. Archives of Neurology 52:754–762.

Schwertner RM, Pinkston D, O'Sullivan P, & Denton B (1987). Transition from student to physical therapist: Changes in perceptions of professional role and relationship between perceptions and job satisfaction. Physical Therapy 67(5): 695–701.

Seibert JH, Brien JS, Maaske BL, Kochurka K, Feldt K, Fader L, & Race KE (1999). Assessing patient satisfaction across the continuum of ambulatory care: A revalidation and validation of care-specific surveys. Journal of Ambulatory Care Management 22(2):9–26.

Sherbourne CD, Sturm R, & Wells KB (1999). What outcomes matter to patients? Journal of General Internal Medicine 14:357–363.

Stewart AL, Hays RD, & Ware JE (1988). The MOS Short Form General Health Survey: Reliability and validity in a patient population. Medical Care 26:724–732.

Stewart D (1993). Health care delivery system. In DL Stewart & SH Abeln (eds.). Documenting Functional Outcomes in Physical Therapy. St. Louis: Mosby-Year Book.

Sullivan, et al. (2000) The relationship of lumbar flexion to disability in patients with low back pain. Physical Therapy 80:240–250.

Teschendorf B & Nemshick M (2001). Faculty roles in professional socialization. Journal of Physical Therapy Education 15(1):4–10.

Testa MA & Nackley JF (1994). Methods for quality of life studies. Annual Review of Public Health 15:535–559.

Turner PA, Harby-Owren H, Shackleford F, So A, Fosse R, & Whitfield TWA (1999). Audits of physiotherapy practice. Physiotherapy Theory and Practice. 15:261–274.

Van den Hout WB, de Jong Z, Munneke M, Hazes JM, Breedveld FC, & Vliet Vlieland TP (2005). Cost-utility and cost-effectiveness analyses of a long-term, high-intensity exercise program compared with conventional physical therapy in patients with rheumatoid arthritis. Arthritis & Rheumatism 53(1):39–47.

Whetten-Goldstein K, Cutson T, Zhu C, & Schenkman M (2000). Financial burden of chronic neurological disorders to patients and their families: What providers need to know. Neurology Report 24 (4):140–144.

.

Consumers of Outcome Data

KEY TERMS

Patient

Clinical settings

Family

Health-care agencies

Special interest groups

Professional associations

Work/community groups

Government

Service providers

Business/industry

CHAPTER OUTCOMES

➤ Identify consumers of outcome data.

➤ Explain how different consumers have different needs for outcome data.

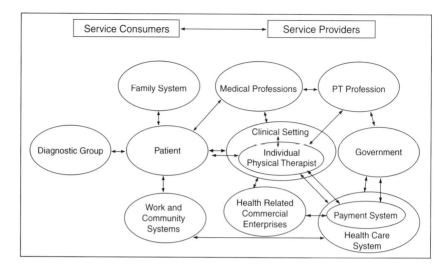

Figure 4.1 Perspectives on outcomes.

A variety of people and institutions have expressed a need for outcome data. Each group has a different perspective as to which data are meaningful and how to apply those data to fit their needs. Despite having separate needs for and interests in outcome data, all of the parties involved in health-care delivery are interconnected. Therefore, meaningful outcomes for one party are influenced by the perspectives and needs of other parties. As the outcomes from a single encounter or episode of intervention can be meaningful to many parties, it is helpful to understand who the parties are and how their perspectives differ.

Figure 4.1 depicts the different parties that are interested in outcome data. In general, the bubbles toward the left side represent the consumers of health-care services, and the bubbles toward the right side represent those that deliver or support health-care services. Each party will be described; sample outcome questions are posed at the end of each section to indicate how that group might pose a question. "Intervention A" will be the imaginary focus of the questions—it represents any intervention or service that a physical therapist or clinic might offer.

THE CONSUMERS

Patients and Clients

Patients and clients who receive physical therapy services are consumers of rehabilitation outcome data. Their interest is at a personal level because they are interested in their own progress relative to their prognosis for improvement. In an outcome approach to care, patients participate in determining meaningful outcomes for intervention. Improved scores on meaningful functional outcomes are important patient indicators that an intervention plan is working. Whereas feedback about changes in impairments may be helpful when appreciable changes in functional limitations have not yet occurred, patients will more clearly see the benefits of physical therapy when functional losses are resolved. Grimmer, et al. (1999) demonstrate that naive patients (those receiving intervention for low back pain for the first time) expect different outcomes of their first intervention session than do experienced patients (those who have received intervention for the same diagnosis in the past). Both groups of patients expect symptom relief, but experienced patients expect more advice and explanation than the naive group. Grimmer, et al. also demonstrate that some expectations can be clearly described by the patient, and some are more covertly assumed. For instance, these researchers found that the decision to return for a second visit was partly influenced by whether patients received symptom relief as well as by the interpersonal skills and ability to provide information of the physical therapists.

From a broader perspective, patients have increasingly more access to medical and technical information to help them manage their health issues. Patients are using the Internet to seek information about physical illness, nutrition, health-care providers or institutions, and alternative treatments (Dickerson, et al., 2004). They seek this information both directly through family or computers and indirectly by having someone who is more comfortable with technology assist them in finding information (Dickerson, et al., 2004; Lea, Lockwood, & Ringash, 2005). Although level of education appears to be a strong predictor of who will access health information on the Internet (Meischke, et al., 2005), the Internet is a growing medium that may influence patients' knowledge about their conditions and expectations for care.

In summary, patients may be able to identify their expected outcomes of intervention when it is related to their condition, but as Grimmer, et al. suggest, there may also be covert expectations that influence patient compliance with a suggested plan of care.

> *A patient will ask, "How will I benefit from intervention?"*

Family and Friends

Family and friends are the people who interact daily with a patient and who may be providers of physical, emotional, or financial support. When a person's level of disability requires intervention, family and friends are also affected (Abramson, et al., 1993). If the patient can no longer perform his or her role of spouse, caregiver, or wage earner, the balance in the family or friendship is altered. Other people may need to assume the patient's prior roles or assist the patient by performing new roles (Whetten-Goldstein, et al., 2000). Family and friends' perceptions of a patient's ability complements the response of a patient who is in denial, who unrealistically assesses function, or who exaggerates reports to cover for feelings of embarrassment or inadequacy (Kessler & Mroczek, 1995; Knapp & Hewison, 1999; Purtillo & Haddad, 1996).

Family structures change over time, and expected outcomes may change as well. When an acute disability becomes chronic, the family is affected by many variables, including the prognosis, personality traits, motivation, economics, communication patterns, and the numbers of members in the immediate and extended support systems. Initially, the family's interest may be in the outcomes of medical management. As time passes, the focus may need to shift to lifestyle adaptations and long-range planning. Swoboda and Lipsett (2002) demonstrate significant burdens on families caring for patients, including loss of employment, stress-related illnesses, economic loss including bankruptcy, and postponement of education.

The outcomes desired by family and friends may not always match the outcomes desired by the patient. For instance, a patient may consider the optimal outcome as returning home where family can assist the patient. In contrast, the family may see the optimal outcome as the patient's placement in a facility where others give the care, because the family perceives barriers to its own abilities to provide satisfactory care. Mismatched expectations are affected by a variety of issues beyond the control of physical therapists, such as cultural values, financial concerns, and the proximity of family members. Nonetheless, the clinician may need to assist the patient and the family in finding a common outcome that both parties can support.

Families are similar to patients in their use of literature or interest in the details of specific outcome studies. They are more likely to use medical professionals as their source of information, supported by information from the lay press and public media. The data that families use are similar to those of patients. Results of periodic examinations and subjective observations about the patient's function combine to influence their decision making.

> *A family might ask, "How much recovery of function do patients with this diagnosis achieve initially and after 5 years?" or "How will intervention help this family member recover function?"*

Special Interest Groups

Special interest groups and support services for specific diagnostic groupings (e.g., the Arthritis Foundation for patients with different types of arthritis) are interested in trends in intervention outcomes. Whereas their services support individual patients and their family systems, the groups and services are interested in outcome data based on larger samples of people with similar diagnoses or levels of disability. Understanding the effectiveness of different types of interventions helps organizations to make budgetary decisions about the services and research they support as well as assist in their ability to disseminate the latest information. For example, the Science & Professional page on the website of the American Heart Association (americanheart.org) provides statistics about the incidence of strokes, cardiovascular disease, and cholesterol studies. The website for the Arthritis Foundation (arthritis.org) posts research results about a variety of conditions, including lupus, arthritis, juvenile arthritis, and irritable bowel disease.

> *Special interest groups might ask, "What percentage of people with this diagnosis is positively affected by intervention A?"*

Work and Community Groups

Patients are part of larger social systems including work and community systems. Successful return to those social systems depends in part on the accessibility of the environments and the accommodations that can be made for a patient. Increasingly, work environments are using prevention programs to minimize the risk of work-related disability. For example, Goodman, et al. (2005) report that 1 year after the implementation of ergonomic principles at computer workstations as taught by a physical and an occupational therapist, an engineering firm saw a reduction of 81% of the original physical problems reported by employees.

Employers use outcome data to support managerial decisions about injury prevention programs and about the benefits they provide to staff. They may also use outcome data to justify preserving, retraining, or replacing an employee who becomes injured. Companies use outcome data to evaluate the benefits they offer to employees. Some of the successful efforts that have occurred in companies include prevention and safety programs, employee health education programs, preventive exercise programs, and even day-care center services (Erben, Franzkowiak, & Wenzel, 1992). Positive cost-benefit outcomes that have been realized include less injury on the job, less absenteeism, and greater morale and productivity (Wynn, 1996).

Communities can be described as private or public, local or statewide. A private community can be small (e.g., a residential center) or large (e.g., a condominium association for healthy elderly people). Public communities include townships and counties, and state borders define statewide communities. No matter what the size is, all have responsibility for addressing the needs of their residents (Epstein & McGee, 1996). Communities use outcome data to predict and address the social, economic, and medical needs of the resident population. The New York City Department of Health (NYC-DOH) is an example of one community's successful use of outcome data to create a strategic community plan in their approach to childhood asthma. In 1996, the NYCDOH Childhood Asthma Initiative was started to improve control and prevention of asthma and to reduce asthma-related hospitalizations. Data demonstrating a 22% increase in asthma-related hospitalizations, with 60% of those coming from low-income families, spurred the implementation of programs to track people with asthma, increase community awareness, promote family management of asthma, and reduce triggers in the environment (NYCDOH, 1999). Since school nurses began teaching an asthma management curriculum to third-graders, the preliminary NYCDOH data indicate a 13% reduction in asthma-related school absences (NYCDOH, 2000).

> *Work settings might ask, "How likely is it that intervention A will allow this employee to return to work?" A community might ask, "Based on census data, how many of our residents might need intervention A, and are we in a position to provide it?"*

THE PROVIDERS

Individual Service Providers

Health-care service providers use outcome data for several purposes. Data from an individual patient serve as a baseline for comparison of progress for that particular patient. This use of outcome data is important for advancing patients towards their goals, but it is limited to the individual patient-clinician relationship.

Data from groups of patients can describe a clinician's general effectiveness with patients having similar problems, a clinician's cost of providing services, the frequencies of interventions provided, or the satisfaction that patients derive from working with a clinician. This information may be use-

> ➤ *Clinicians use outcome data to:*
> - *Describe clinician effectiveness with patients.*
> - *Advocate for patient management strategies.*
> - *Reflect on practice trends.*
> - *Compare their results with those of other clinicians.*

ful for describing intervention strategies, identifying best clinical practice patterns, identifying education needs, determining supply and equipment needs, or clarifying strengths and weaknesses perceived by patients relative to a clinician's service delivery. Data describing the course of similar injuries or problems can help a clinician predict and negotiate expected outcomes and develop clinical pathways or preferred service procedures.

An increasing role for clinicians is that of patient advocate and financial manager. Accurate patient data sets can yield descriptions of the percentage of patients who have been successfully assisted to a particular level of independence. This type of data analysis can be instrumental in convincing third-party payers to approve a plan of intervention that may be different from what is typically covered. For instance, a clinician might want to schedule a patient's limited visits over 4 months but finds that the patient's insurance benefits cover services rendered for only the first 2 months. A claims reviewer might be more inclined to grant an exception for 2 visits per week for 4 months rather than pay for 4 visits a week for 2 months if the clinician has data to show that patients with similar problems typically require a full 4 months to regain the functional levels required for a full return to work. When these data are combined with published studies, the appeal can be quite convincing.

Clinicians can also benefit from accurate data about their practice to develop their own personal report cards. The reflective clinician is one who assesses prior practice to inform future clinical decisions. Outcome data on the patients treated by a single clinician provide that clinician with objective measures of success and thus eliminate the reliance on intuition.

Clinicians can also use outcome data for comparison with other clinicians treating the same diagnostic groups. Improving individual approaches to patients, developing the most effective intervention methods, and then sharing successes with colleagues through informal and formal presentations have a rich tradition in the medical community. As with any other comparison, the ability to compare one clinician's approach with that of another is greatly increased when the descriptions of what has been done is defined well and measured objectively.

> *A provider might ask, "What are the characteristics of my patients who have responded best to intervention A versus those who do not respond at all?" or "How successful am I in reaching functional goals for patients receiving intervention A?"*

Clinical Settings

The clinical setting is the business structure that provides health-care services. A hospital may have a rehabilitation department that provides inpatient and outpatient services. A home health agency may send individual service providers into skilled nursing facilities or patients' homes. A public school system may have a staff of clinicians who provide services in schools within the district. Whatever the venue of service provision, administrative planning, accountability, and patient service delivery can be supported and guided by outcome data.

Clinical settings are interested in outcome data that reflect larger numbers of patients and broader issues of service delivery. As described in

Chapter 3, some of the more common outcome interests include patient satisfaction, cost of services, and intervention effectiveness across different settings. For example, Kramer, et al. (2003) compare impairment and functional outcomes of 160 patients who had unilateral total knee arthroplasties and who were treated in either outpatient clinics or through home-based exercise programs with telephone follow-ups. Areas that are less often studied are clinician outcomes, which include comparisons of clinicians' effectiveness with patients, clinicians' costs of providing services, and clinicians' satisfaction with professional responsibilities.

> *A clinical setting's administration might ask, "How often is intervention A used by our clinicians, and how does use relate to the time until discharge, the number of patient visits, or the functional levels achieved by patients?" or "What are the costs associated with intervention A versus those of intervention B, and how do they relate to patient outcomes?"*

Health Care and Reimbursement Agencies

Government agencies and private insurance programs rely heavily on outcome data (or their absence) to make management and policy decisions (Hebbeler, 2004; Mariner, 1994). Justification for provision of service has more recently been linked to documented effectiveness because the companies are liable for the services they provide. Managed care organizations, by the nature of their intent to manage a patient's care plan, are responsible for providing appropriate services and for protecting their customers from harmful interventions (Bailit, Federico, & McGivney, 1995). Decisions whether to cover certain types of interventions are based on a thorough review process when possible, but public and political opinion can influence that process. Recent examples of practices affected by data and public opinion include the increased duration of maternal stay following delivery (Eaton, 2001; Madden, et al., 2003), decisions about which complementary and alternative medicine approaches to cover (Pelletier, Astin, & Haskell, 1999), and decisions about reimbursement for brand name pharmaceuticals versus generic products (Suh, 1999).

The viewpoint that health-care and reimbursement agencies bring to outcome data is very different from the interests of clinicians and patients. Bailit, Federico, and McGivney (1995) describe five steps that insurers use to assess the effectiveness of an intervention.

The first step is *issue identification,* when interventions with undetermined effectiveness are identified. Medical administrators may identify interventions because customers are requesting reimbursement for them, or they arise in the literature or medical community as a new way to treat a particular health problem, or they become a priority because of their cost or the number of people that might use them.

The second step is the *evaluation* of an intervention on the priority list. Previously published data and new data from scientific studies of the intervention's outcomes are reviewed. Based on these data and a formal evaluation, a *medical assessment* is made about the intervention's usefulness. Medical panels, business administrators, and legal advisors review the assessment before a *coverage policy* is formulated. The fifth step is the *dis-*

semination of the policy to claims-processing and utilization review centers and possibly to medical journals for publication of the evaluation study for further public scrutiny.

It is important for service providers to understand the processes that companies undertake when determining the effectiveness of interventions and thus how a decision to reimburse for them is made. For example, beginning with issue identification, a company might discover many of the interventions used by physical therapists have not undergone rigorous outcome studies to clearly demonstrate their effectiveness; others may not have been studied at all. From an insurer's perspective, the process would probably generate a long list of issues, resulting in one of two policy decisions. The first decision might be that as the intervention has not been studied enough to indicate its effectiveness, it need not be offered as a reimbursable service. The alternate conclusion might be that the intervention has been commonly accepted, despite a lack of support, so reimbursement may be approved. Although an individual service provider may be adamant that an intervention is effective for a particular patient and assert that the intervention is a well-accepted intervention in professional practice, insurers are not likely to create coverage policies based on the experience of individual providers.

The confusion for individual service providers may increase when reimbursement has been given in the past from the same company, other companies reimburse for it, or individual claims processors give isolated approvals for it (Bailit, Federico, & McGivney, 1995). In these situations, careful documentation of the patient's impairment and functional status as well as logical communication about the relationship of the intervention to functional outcomes may be the basis for individual decisions to cover the intervention. These case-by-case decisions are not the same as reimbursement decisions based on a company policy that establishes guidelines for the intervention and its reimbursement.

Another perspective that health-care organizations and insurers brings to the use of outcome data is their role in the contractual relationship they have with each patient. This relationship is defined only by agreement between the parties to the services or products outlined in the insurance policy. The offering party (i.e., the insurer) is held to state and federal legal standards but is not generally held to moral or ethical standards in the way that health-care providers are. Thus, an organization sees itself as accountable if it upholds the agreements and obligations it has made with its customers (the patients), and customers are encouraged to "shop around" to purchase the best insurance service their money can buy.

In contrast, health-care providers are governed by state and federal legal standards and also answer to ethical or professional standards relative to the quality of care delivered and the demonstration of compassionate care (Banja & Johnston, 1994). This is an essential difference in perspective that drives how decisions to provide care and associated reimbursements are made. A conflict might arise when a clinician offers a service that an organization or insurer does not cover and the patient does not have the financial means to purchase the service directly.

There are factors independent of patients that influence how an insurer creates an insurance coverage product. One factor is customer competition. The ability to offer the types and amounts of services that the public is seeking at a more competitive price can be achieved by mixing different coverage options together or by restricting access to selected health-care providers. If competing insurers are selling plans that include other types of coverage, a company would need to assess its own ability to offer that service just to maintain its fair share of the marketplace. This creates a form of peer pressure from within the industry that is also responsive to public opinion and demand as well as outcome data from professional organizations.

The decision not to cover certain types of services can also lead to lawsuits or poor publicity from customers or service providers, and this factor affects what may or may not be offered to patients. The expenses of dealing with lawsuits and reversing public opinion about a company's policies may equal or overshadow the actual reimbursement expenses to make that coverage available. Loss of market share (a business outcome) due to poor publicity over policies or lawsuits can be a very strong factor in determining what the insurer provides (Bailit, Federico, & McGivney, 1995).

> *Health-care agencies and insurers might ask, "How often are we billed for intervention A, and is there documentation to support continued reimbursement?"*

Professional Associations

Professional associations serve many functions and constituents. One function they perform is defining a scope of practice relative to other professions and policy makers. This is done in part by documenting what its members do and organizing evidence for the profession's effectiveness. In physical therapy, the focus is on describing the settings that provide services, the patients and communities that are served, the clinical decision-making processes that are used to provide interventions, and to the effectiveness of those interventions to the public. Professional associations support outcome research through the funding of publications and educational and research opportunities (Benjamin, 1995). Professional associations encourage outcome studies to develop clinical pathways and practice guidelines, to support the use and reimbursement for preferred practice patterns (Mariner, 1994), and to influence policy development (Benjamin, 1995; Benjamin, Perfetto, & Greene, 1995).

> *A professional association might ask, "Is there adequate, documented evidence for the use of intervention A and, if not, should we fund studies to examine it more carefully?"*

Government

Government agencies set policies at all levels that directly affect the provision of health care. In 1989, the Patient Outcome Research Act was passed by Congress to establish a patient-centered outcome research program (Ware, 1995). In 1989, the Agency for Health Care Policy and Research (AHCPR) was created to disseminate information and organize outcome research (ahcpr.gov/about/profile.htm; Mariner, 1994). In 1999, the government reauthorized the AHCPR under a new name, the Agency for Healthcare Research and Quality (AHRQ), with the mission of supporting research to improve health care (ahcpr.gov/about/profile.htm). An agenda called Healthy People 2000 was established to address prevention of disease and disability and health-related quality of life (HRQOL). In order to track data related to

HRQOL on a state level, federal support to establish a surveillance tool was channeled through the Centers for Disease Control's National Center for Chronic Disease Prevention and Health Promotion in 1991–1992 (Hennessy, et al., 1994). A series of expert discussions resulted in the adoption of four key questions that described HRQOL, which were added to the 1993 Behavioral Risk Factor Surveillance System survey. This telephone survey was administered to over 100,000 people in 49 states (Hennessy, et al., 1994). Additional efforts to collect HRQOL data include such studies as the annual National Health Interview Survey (Connell, Diehr, & Hart, 1987; Hennessy, et al., 1994); the Health Employers Data and Information Set (HEDIS), which is generated by managed care plans (Epstein & McGee, 1996); and NIH-sponsored clinical trials that must now address general functional outcomes as well as disease or organ-related outcomes (Ware, 1995).

As the single largest payer for health care, the federal government supports the study of health-care standards, health-care plans, and consumer education efforts. Data are collected from a variety of health-care delivery settings such as hospitals, nursing facilities, ambulatory care centers, and home health agencies (Epstein & McGee, 1996). Thirty-eight states have initiatives to collect, analyze, and disseminate health-care data, however, these initiatives are subject to changes due to funding and election results (Epstein & McGee, 1996). Several states publish performance report cards on the outcomes of care by the type of provider, patient diagnosis, and medical procedure (Royal & Bueno, 1999). Despite the variability in efforts, it is clear that government agencies at both the state and federal levels are interested in health and health services outcomes in order to determine the effectiveness of care, to determine standards of patient care and provider education, to influence cost control, and to identify the services or products that should be reimbursed by government sponsored health-care plans (Benjamin, Perfetto, & Greene, 1995; Mariner, 1994).

> A government agency might ask "Are the studies available on intervention A extensive and valid enough to understand its place in clinical guidelines?"

Other Medical Professions

Patients seek and receive health-care interventions from many different sources. Given the restructuring of health-care delivery systems and reimbursement practices, every type of health-care provider is being pressed to evaluate the effectiveness of its services and improve accountability on many levels. Measurement of outcomes is occurring in all areas; from short- and long-term intervention efficacy to service delivery efficiency and patient satisfaction. Each profession is struggling with how to integrate data that are important within its field with those of other service providers and regulatory agencies.

The questions that each professional group must address are similar. Among those questions are such global issues as how to introduce the need for outcome measures to its clinicians, how best to collect data, how to identify meaningful outcome measures when more than one discipline is responsible for patient care, and how to describe how outcomes affect practice guidelines. This is evidenced in the types of articles that appear in discipline-specific journals. In the *Archives of Internal Medicine,* Woolf (1993) writes about the impact of practice guidelines on patient care. Wiley in *Rehabilitation Management* (1993) describes the reasons for and the types of data physical therapists are trying to collect. Crawford, et al. (1996) argue in the *Journal of Nursing Care Quality* that the nursing perspective has been left out of physician-directed studies and offers suggestions for less traditional patient outcome measures. Finally, in the *Journal of Substance Abuse Treatment,* Desmond, et al. (1995) describe methods to improve long-term follow-up of psychiatric outcomes on patients who were treated for substance abuse.

Physical therapists use outcome studies from a variety of professions to assist with clinical decision-making processes. More and more, as physical therapists and physicians collaboratively manage patients to achieve optimal HRQOL, outcome data from a variety of professions are shared.

> *Other health-care providers might ask, "What is intervention A, and how might it affect what I am doing with a particular patient?"*

Business and Industry

The provision of health care is supported by many businesses. These include businesses that develop and produce durable and consumable medical products, support services for management such as software programs, documentation and billing technology, transportation services, educational services, and publishers of health-care–related books and journals. Managed care and cost-containment practices are driving the medical products industry to become more accountable for identifying the cost benefits of new products relative to what currently exists (Last & Nash, 1995; Williams, 1991).

Cost comparison studies for specific products and for the overall management of a patient have become especially valued by reimbursement agencies. For example, demonstrating that a new product costs the same but lasts twice as long as a previously existing product would support a reimbursement policy to cover the new product. Likewise, identifying an intervention that may cost more initially but that might decrease the average overall hospital stay of the typical patient would also support the decision to reimburse for the newer, more expensive product.

The process that industry must use to produce useful outcome data combines the measurement of patient-related outcomes, service outcomes, and cost outcomes. These outcomes include the patients' responses to intervention, mortality and morbidity outcomes, and data on costs associated with interventions. Clinical trials have long been a standard for establishing efficacy of interventions; only recently have broader issues of patient satisfaction with a product and improvements in quality of life been included in those assessments (Ware, 1995). After being collected, the data are merged to identify the cost-effectiveness of a particular product or intervention. Once that cost-effectiveness is established, it can be marketed to the medical community or general public (Last & Nash, 1995). An example of a comparison of two services is provided in a study by Indredavik, et al. (1998). In a randomized controlled clinical trial, they demonstrate that patients who received specialized stroke unit care for a first infarct had greater function and HRQOL scores 5 years later than those receiving general hospital care.

Business and industry might ask, "How will this new product (intervention A) affect the overall cost of management of a patient relative to intervention B?" or "Will this new product (intervention A) significantly improve the overall function and patient quality of life relative to a currently existing product, even if it costs more than the old product?"

INTEGRATING DIFFERENT PERSPECTIVES IN OUTCOME DATA

Different Perspectives Influence the Question Studied

When beginning a study, it is important to identify which perspective is being addressed. Each perspective has a different way of framing a research question and using the available outcome data (Luce & Simpson, 1995). For example, a meaningful rehabilitation outcome for a patient may be to progress from using a walker to using a standard cane. This outcome is directly affected by the patient's financial support, the family requirements for the patient's independence, the period for rehabilitation, and the clinician's competence in assessing the potential for achieving that goal. A family that can provide assistance in achieving the goal may accelerate the patient's process, whereas a patient with a family that cannot help may require more time, a different strategy for achieving the goal, or a choice of a different goal. The experience level of the clinician may influence the patient's outcome depending on how conservatively or aggressively the patient is managed. The outcomes are important to the patient, and the other parties in the health-care delivery system affect the patient's ability to achieve those outcomes.

From a different perspective, the achievement of walking with a standard cane will be of interest to the individual physical therapist. Depending on the severity of the patient's diagnosis, the goal may be considered a typical and routine goal; however, if the patient is not progressing after the first week or so, the clinician may need to question the effectiveness of the intervention approach or the importance of that goal to the patient. From the clinician's perspective, the outcome is a measure of intervention effectiveness.

Managers of physical therapy services might be interested in the cost-efficiency of providing services to reach the goal. A manager might question whether the physical therapist needs to render all of the service and what roles exist for physical therapist assistants or aides.

Another perspective on the same goal comes from the third-party payer. A claims reviewer might ask whether there is any functional benefit from achieving the goal and, if so, what is the typical number of visits to achieve it. Third-party payers are becoming more selective about the amount of physical therapy they will provide and look at the cost-benefit of getting a patient to a particular level of function.

Thus, data on the goal for the patient can be viewed from many perspectives. When creating data sets on similar patients, the investigating clinician will want to identify who will be using the data and what type of reports might be helpful to generate.

Different Perspectives May Influence How Results Are Explained

When interpreting outcome data for others to digest, it is important to understand the audience's perspective. Obvious audiences for outcome data are colleagues in similar practices and service providers from the continuum of care that flanks a practice. In the first case, colleagues in similar practice settings are seeing some of the same types of patients and would be interested in what has been found. In the second case, clinical settings that precede or follow a particular type of service in the continuum of care might benefit from outcome data that describes patients at the start or end of services.

Although the intent of most outcome studies is ultimately to improve practice or service delivery, it is possible to misinterpret data or not interpret them fully enough for readers from other professions or perspectives to appreciate the contributions that are made. Care must be taken to understand who will be viewing the data and whether they are ready for public consumption. This is presented in Chapter 12 with greater depth.

SUMMARY

Technical and scientific advances in medical and rehabilitation management occur rapidly and constantly. This rapid change requires that all consumers and providers of health-care services (see Fig. 4.1) continually update their understandings about the expected outcomes of health-care services. For the providers of health-care services, this means reading what has been done by others with regard to a new intervention and monitoring patient care for intervention effectiveness. Regardless of the role in service delivery, clinicians should appreciate that the patient bubble appears in every discussion. Outcome data reflect the experience of the patient in relation to all of the other parties; without the patient, the other parties have no role.

In addition, both consumers and providers are connected by a single purpose: the delivery of health care to the patient. Changes made in one bubble affect decisions and service delivery in many other bubbles and ultimately affect the patient. Policy makers and insurers may need to review the effectiveness of new interventions to determine safety regulations, practice act limitations, and reimbursement policies. Their determinations can directly influence the denial or approval of coverage or changes in access to a new intervention, which directly affects each patient who may benefit from the intervention. Conversely, as the number and average age of patients increase, the cost of maintaining good health and managing more complicated chronic conditions increases. These economic strains affect the insurers who must make decisions about the health-care plans they can offer.

All of the parties are influenced by public acceptance of interventions, the strength of related outcome studies, the social and political agendas of the time, cultural and ethical values, and changing economics. This interconnectedness accounts for the widespread request for outcome measures and the overall confusion about what outcome measures to produce. Every party has slightly different needs for information, and yet all parties need some of the same information.

References

Abramson JS, Donnelly J, King MA, & Mailick MD (1993). Disagreements in discharge planning: A normative phenomenon. Health & Social Work 18(1):57–64.

Bailit H, Federico J, & McGivney W (1995). Use of outcomes studies by a managed care organization: Valuing measured treatment effects. Medical Care 33(4) AS216-AS225.

Banja J & Johnston MV (1994). Outcomes evaluation in TBI rehabilitation. Part III: Ethical perspectives and social policy. Archives of Physical Medicine and Rehabilitation 75:SC19-SC26.

Benjamin K (1995). Outcomes research and the allied health professional. Journal of Allied Health. 24(1)3–12.

Benjamin KL, Perfetto EM, & Greene RJ (1995). Public policy and the application of outcomes assessment paradigms versus politics. Medical Care 33(4):AS299–AS306.

Connell FA, Diehr P, & Hart LG (1987). The use of large data bases in health care studies. Annual Reviews in Public Health 8:51–74.

Crawford BL, Taylor LS, Seipert BS, & Lush M (1996). The imperative of outcomes analysis: An integration of traditional and nontraditional outcomes measures. Journal of Nursing Care Quality 10(2):33–40.

Desmond DP, Maddux JF, Johnson TH, & Confer BA (1995). Obtaining follow-up interviews for treatment evaluation. Journal of Substance Abuse Treatment 12(2):95–102.

Dickerson S, Reinhart AM, Feeley TH, Bidani R, Rich E, Garg VK, & Hershey C (2004). Patient Internet use for health information at three urban primary care clinics. Journal of American Medical Informatics Association 11(6):499–504.

Eaton AP (2001). Early postpartum discharge: Recommendations from a preliminary report to Congress. Pediatrics 107:400–403.

Epstein MH & McGee JL (1996). Roles of the federal and state governments in outcomes assessment. American Journal of Medical Quality 11(1):S18–S21.

Erben R, Franzkowiak P, & Wenzel E (1992). Assessment of the outcomes of health intervention. Social Science and Medicine 35(4):359–365.

Goodman G, Landis J, George C, McGuire S, Shorter C, Sieminski M, & Wilson T (2005). Effectiveness of computer ergonomics interventions for an engineering company: A program evaluation. WORK: A Journal of Prevention, Assessment & Rehabilitation 24(1):53–62.

Grimmer K, Sheppard L, Pitt M, Magarey M, & Trott P (1999). Differences in stakeholder expectations in the outcome of physiotherapy management of acute low back pain. International Society for Quality in Health Care 11(2):155–162.

Hebbeler K (2004). Uses and misuses of data on outcome for young children with disabilities (Draft). Early Childhood Outcomes Center, US Office of Special Education Programs. fpg.unc.edu/~ECO/pdfs/ECO_Outcomes_Uses.pdf

Hennessy CH, Moriarty DG, Zack MM, Scherr PA, & Brackbill R (1994). Measuring health-related quality of life for public health surveillance. Public Health Reports 109(5):665–672.

Indredavik B, Bakke F, Slordahl SA, Rokseth R, & Haheim LL (1998). Stroke unit treatment improves long-term quality of life: A randomized controlled trial. Stroke 29:895–899.

Kessler RC & Mroczek DK (1995). Measuring the effects of medical interventions. Medical Care 33(4):AS109-AS119.

Knapp P & Hewison J (1999). Disagreement in patient and career assessment of functional capabilities after stroke. Stroke 30:934–938.

Kramer JF, Speechley M, Bourne R, Rorabeck C, & Vaz M (2003). Comparison of clinic- and home-based rehabilitation programs after total knee arthroplasty. Clinical Orthopaedics and Related Research 410:225–234.

Last JV & Nash DB (1995). Developing health care products in a managed care environment. The Journal of Outcomes Management 2(1):18–21.

Lea J, Lockwood G, & Ringash J (2005). Survey of computer use for health topics by patients with head and neck cancer. Head & Neck 27:8–14.

Luce BR & Simpson K (1995). Methods of cost-effectiveness analysis: Areas of consensus and debate. Clinical Therapeutics 17(1):109–125.

Madden JM, Soumerai SB, Lieu TA, Mandl KD, Zhang F, & Ross-Degnan D (2003). Effects of a law against early postpartum discharge on newborn follow-up, adverse events, and HMO expenditures. New England Journal of Medicine 347(25):2031–2038.

Mariner WK (1994). Outcomes assessment in health care reform: Promise and limitations. American Journal of Law and Medicine, 20 (1,2):37–57.

Meischke H, Eisenberg M, Rowe S, & Cagle A (2005). Do older adults use the Internet for information on heart attacks? Results from a survey of seniors in King County, Washington. Heart Lung 34:3–12.

New York City Department of Health (1999). Asthma Facts. Community Healthworks. New York City.

New York City Department of Health (2000). Open Airways for Schools. School Health Program, New York City.

Pelletier KR, Astin JA, & Haskell WL.(1999). Current trends in the integration and reimbursement of complementary and alternative medicine by managed care organizations (MCOs) and insurance providers: 1998 update and cohort analysis. American Journal of Health Promotion 14(2):125–133.

Purtillo R & Haddad A (1996). Challenges to patients. In Health Professional and Patient Interaction, pp 117–135. Philadelphia: W.B. Saunders Co.

Royal N & Bueno M (1999). Improving performance though change: An academic medical center's experience. Nursing Administration Quarterly 23(2):74–82.

Suh DC (1999). Trends of generic substitution in community pharmacies. Pharmacy World & Science 21(6):260–265.

Swoboda SM & Lipsett PA (2002). Impact of a prolonged surgical critical illness on patients' families. American Journal of Critical Care 11(5):459–466.

Ware, JE (1995). The status of health assessment. Annual Reviews in Public Health 16:327–354.

Whetten-Goldstein K, Cutson T, Zhu C, & Schenkman M (2000). Financial burden of chronic neurological disorders to patients and their families: What providers need to know. Neurology Report 24(4):140–144.

Wiley G (1993). A scramble for facts. Rehabilitation Management June/July:165–167.

Williams A (1991). The role of health economics in clinical decision-making: Is it ethical? Respiratory Medicine 85(Supplement B):3–5.

Woolf SH (1993). Practice guidelines: A new reality in medicine. Part III: Impact on patient care. Archives of Internal Medicine 153:2646–2655.

Wynn, KE (1996). Setting corporate trends with on-site PT. PT Magazine 4(7):66–71.

Models of Disablement

Designing an outcome study is easier if the clinician has a way to organize observations and hypotheses about those observations. Theories and models help to describe hypothesized relationships among observations or constructs. In all systematic inquiry, a description of the theory or model that is being tested is useful for interpreting the data analysis. This chapter describes what a model is, reviews the variety of disablement models that appear in the physical therapy literature, and highlights the challenges in integrating theories with clinical practice and research.

THEORIES AND MODELS

Theories describe *relationships* among concepts, structures, or phenomena. A model is a *graphic or physical representation* of a theory. It might represent the orientation of physical elements (such as a model of a carbon molecule), the relationship of concepts (such as a food pyramid), or the order of a process (such as the Krebs cycle). Theories help to organize and explain observations; models provide a visual representation of relationships.

> *Models are graphic descriptions of relationships.*

Models also provide categories for classifying observations. Each section of a model is operationally defined, such that each section or part is mutually exclusive of other parts. Operational definitions define categories and variables for their unique applications in a study (Portney & Watkins, 2000) and allow the user to sort information into the appropriate parts of a model. For example, the Nagi Model of Disablement has four parts: pathology impairments, functional limitations, and disabilities. Patient problems can be classified according to the operational definitions for this model, and theories about the relationship of impairments to functional limitations or disabilities can be generated and tested through intervention.

> *Models provide structure for classification of observations.*

> *Models provide a common language across settings.*

Models allow users to speak the same language and to classify information in the same way across many settings. When clinicians agree to use a specific model, they are agreeing to use the operational definitions as created by the originator of the model. By using the same definitions of terms, the observations, processes, or events unique to one setting or patient can be combined or compared with those from other clinicians or settings.

MODELS OF DISABLEMENT

Several models of disablement have been created to describe the relationship of disease or injury to the consequences of the disease or injury. These models are presented to highlight the differences in terminology that are used to describe the disablement process; in some cases, the same word is found in different models and defines very different concepts. There is no international agreement on which model or set of terminology is acceptable, so clinicians need to be aware of the differences to correctly interpret literature. In addition, the terminology has changed over time. For example, in the Guide to Physical Therapist Practice (2001), the American Physical Therapy Association (APTA) uses language consistent with the Nagi model as a framework for organizing practice descriptions. More recently, the International Classification of Functioning, Disability, and Health (ICF) model has been used as the organizing framework for presentations at the IIISTEP conference (2005), and APTA is collaborating with other disciplines in writing a clinical manual to interpret the ICF for practice (APTA, 2005).

Table 5.1

Classification Schema					
Source	System	Body	Task	Context	Social/Roles
National Center for Medical Rehabilitation Research US Dept. of Health and Human Services (1993)	Pathophysiology	Impairment	Functional limitations	Disability	Societal limitations
International Classification of Impairments, Disabilities, and Handicaps World Health Organization (1980)	Disease	Impairment		Disability	Handicap
ICF World Health Organization (2001)	Disease, disorder, or injury	Body functions/ structures Impairments	Activities Activity limitation	Participation Disability	
Nagi Jette AM (1994).	Active pathology	Impairment	Functional limitations	Disability	
Jette Jette AM (1994).	Pathology	Impairment	Functional limitations Quality of life	Disability	
APTA (2001)	Injury, disease, or other causes	Impairment	Functional limitations	Disability	

In general, disablement models begin with problems at the system or cellular level and progress to problems at the body level, then task level, and finally social/role level. Table 5.1 identifies the more common models and their respective terminology across these categories. The next section provides more detailed descriptions of each category.

The System Level

This category represents the body at the physiological and tissue level. This category identifies the disease process from characteristic changes in cellular physiology and biochemical and anatomical abnormalities (Jette, 1994). In most situations, physical therapists are not diagnosing at the system level. When an initial physical therapy visit reveals a problem at the system level through differential diagnosis, the patient is referred for a medical diagnosis and management, while the physical therapist may or may not continue to address the physical therapy diagnosis at other levels.

The Body Level

This category refers to loss or abnormality at the tissue or organ level resulting in such changes as limited range of motion, decreases in strength or endurance, and postural malalignment. There is agreement across all models in calling these losses *impairments*. This category is frequently studied in physical therapy literature. Changes in range of motion (ROM), strength, and endurance are routinely quantified, and change is relatively easy to report.

The Task Level

A task is a skill that uses a person's available ROM, strength, and coordination to achieve a functional goal. Examples of tasks include rising from a chair, ascending and descending steps, reaching, and walking. The National Center for Medical Rehabilitation Research (NCMRR) and the World Health Organization ICF models separate skill performance from the contexts in which they occur. The NCMRR labels losses of those skills as *functional limitations*. The original version of the International Classification of Impairment, Disability and Handicap (ICIDH) used the term *disability* to describe functional losses (World Health Organization, 1980). In the revision of that document, the ICF has shifted its perspective to focus on the abilities of people. This shift is reflected in the new terminology that uses *activity* to describe performance of tasks and *activity limitation* to describe difficulties with performance of tasks (World Health Organization, 2001).

The Context Level

The context refers to the environment in which a skill is performed. Rising from a chair in a rehabilitation department may be quite different from the transition needed to get out of a car or up from a toilet. When skills cannot be generalized to an environment that is important to the patient, the patient loses access to or independence in those environments. The NCMRR classifies these losses as *disabilities* (US Dept. of HHS, 1993). In the ICF model, environmental factors are classified as *facilitators* or *barriers*.

The Nagi, Jette, and the APTA models do not separate the tasks from the contexts where they occur, although Verbrugge and Jette (1994) propose an adaptation that includes *extra-individual factors* to recognize the role of external supports and the physical environment. In these classification schemas, performances of skills in meaningful contexts are grouped together and are referred to as *functional limitations*. All agree, however, that the limitations are specific to the individual's performance of activities.

The Social/Role Level

This category refers to the roles that people play in their personal and societal lives. Examples include such roles as employer or wage earner, spouse or partner, parent or child, teacher or student. Losses occur when a person is no longer able to fulfill the requirements of a particular role. The NCMRR model identifies these losses as *societal limitations*, the ICIDH called them *handicaps,* the ICF refers to *participation restrictions,* and Nagi, Jette, and APTA models call them *disabilities*. All agree that the limitations are relative to the combined conditions of the individual, the environment, and other people that help to define the individual's roles and participation in society.

THE CONFUSION IN TERMINOLOGY

Table 5.1 illustrates that at the task, context, and social/role levels, identical terms are used to describe different classifications of losses. An *activity limitation* for the ICF is comparable to a *functional limitation* in Nagi's model. Additionally, the same term, *disability,* is called a *handicap* in the original ICIDH model and *participation restriction* in the ICF model. Differences in terminology reflect differences in philosophy, how the models are used, and changes in societal values.

The changes in the social/role category came from sensitivity to language and the implications that certain words carry. The ICIDH (1980) used the term *handicap* in reference to the activities and roles a person cannot perform. Public concern arose from the unfortunate extension of the term to reflect the actual capability of the person. Thus, people were referred to as handicapped rather than referring to the conditions or situations that create a handicap in participation. The World Health Organization has addressed these concerns over language in the ICF. The current categories use both positive and negative terms to describe what a person can and cannot do rather than focus only on their losses.

It is important to appreciate the differences in terminology when reading literature. The reader will need to identify which model the authors are using in order to interpret data or discussions correctly. Authors usually identify their classification schema in the introduction to the article. When comparing studies using different schema, a reader may find it useful to translate studies according to a single model's terminology.

APPLICATION OF DISABLEMENT MODELS TO CLINICAL PRACTICE

Classifying the consequences of illness according to a particular model has many applications to clinical practice. Models of disablement provide frameworks for organizing patient problems, choosing assessments of patient status, choosing interventions, and framing research questions. They provide a common language for describing patient status and for sharing patient information and research data. Finally, they help organize relationships among patient variables that can be tested, accepted, modified, or rejected.

Models Describe Relationships Between Impairments and Function

A model of disablement helps the clinician develop hypotheses about which patient problems might have the greatest impact on patient function. Craik (1994) poses three essential questions:

- What impairments contribute to performance?
- How many of these variables can be modified by treatment?
- If the impairments are modified, is the residual disability reduced?

Patients often have multiple measurable impairments, but not all impairments affect function, nor are all impairments ones that physical therapy can

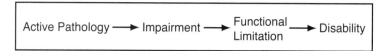

Figure 5.1 Nagi's Model of Disablement. (Adapted from Jette AM [1994]. Physical disablement concepts for physical therapy research and practice. Physical Therapy 74:380–386.)

address. By selecting from a variety of patient and contextual variables, the therapist can design intervention plans that link remediation or adaptation of an impairment with a change in functional performance or disability level. If the intervention is administered, and the expected outcome is achieved, then the therapist has data to support the clinical decision-making process. If the expected outcome is not achieved, the therapist has a framework from which to evaluate the choice of problems to treat, the interventions that were used, and, most important, whether the relationship of the patient problems to the expected outcomes is essentially valid.

➤ *Not all of the patient's physical impairments are related to the functional limitations.*

Linear models of disablement, such as the Nagi model, imply a progression from disease to impairment to functional limitations, which finally result in disability (Fig. 5.1). Although this progression is exhibited in many patients, it should not be assumed that all patients follow this path (Jette, 1995). Patients can present with a wide array of impairments without being functionally or socially limited. For example, a person with cerebral palsy may present with multiple impairments such as limited joint mobility, poor standing balance and reaction times, and diminished ability to generate muscle force. Despite the presence of these impairments, this person can be fully independent in the community by using assistive devices in the home and work environments. Conversely, someone can have significant functional or social limitations without any explicit physical impairment.

➤ *Patients do not always follow a linear progression of disablement.*

The extent of functional limitation is not always proportional to the type and severity of patient impairments. The context in which an activity is performed strongly influences the perceived level of functional limitation (Haley, Coster, & Binda-Sundberg, 1994). The context is a combination of the unique requirements of the activity, personal and environmental expectations of performance, and the cognitive and motivational levels of the person performing. Consider when someone is learning a new sport, such as skiing. Perception of mastery on the beginner's hill can quickly change to one of severe limitation when that person is placed on an advanced racing course.

➤ *Levels of functional limitation are modified by environmental demands.*

When skills are learned or tested out of the context in which they need to be performed, the types of impairments may have less impact on the outcome measurements. This point is nicely illustrated by Doty, et al. (1999) who looked at the performance of ball-handling skills by age-matched children with and without developmental delay. They found that performance of selected skills on standardized tests resulted in higher scores during 1:1 testing than when the skills were observed during a game with peers that required the use of those skills. The level of functional ability that appeared in the isolated testing situation (similar to how physical therapists train or test many patients on safety and mobility skills) was a functional limitation when placed in the social and environmental context in which it was needed.

The ICF model (Fig. 5.2) provides a more dynamic model of the interactions of impairments, functional limitations, and role participation. In this

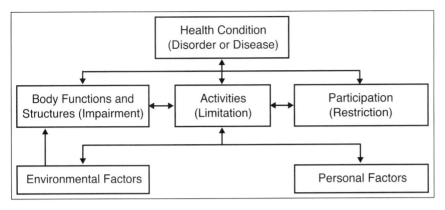

Figure 5.2 The ICF Model of Functioning and Disability. (From International Classification of Functioning, Disability and Health: ICF [2001]. World Health Organization, Geneva, Switzerland.)

model, the arrows are bidirectional, and the impact of the disease and environmental and personal factors are included.

Models Can Help Clinicians to Organize Examinations

When a model of disablement is used to categorize a patient's problems, the clinician can organize tests and measures to reflect the expected changes. When there are limitations at the impairment level, then tests and measures that address the specific impairments may be chosen and documented. When there are limitations at the functional level, tests and measures that quantify changes in functional status are selected. When there are limitations at the social/role level, measures of social and role participation are selected. It is no longer acceptable to document measures of impairments without documenting measures of the function or role that those impairments are believed to effect. In fact, when the goal is to improve function, impairment interventions become strategies to achieve the functional goal rather than the goals themselves.

The challenge that physical therapists face is in identifying the appropriate tests and measures for quantifying function and role participation. There are many more standardized measures of impairment than there are for function or social/role limitations. The number of diagnosis-specific functional and disability assessments are increasingly evident in the literature, and it is the physical therapist's responsibility to search them out and evaluate their usefulness. When standardized assessments are not available, the physical therapist must generate patient-specific measures of change. This is best accomplished by using the functional and role participation goals that the patient has identified as important and, with the patient, establishing a measurement of change that is meaningful in task and context.

Models Help to Organize Plans of Care

Clinicians can use models to organize their patients' plans of care. Nagi's model has four components and, as a consequence of the pathology, a patient may have problems in each component. When a patient presents in a clinical setting, the physical therapist examination generates quantitative data about the impairments, functional losses, and the impact on social roles. The physical therapist diagnosis is the interpretation of that data, including a hypothesis about the relationship of identified impairments and their effects on functional limitations and role participation.

> *The clinical hypothesis drives the selection of interventions.*

The hypothesis about the impact that impairments have on function and role participation is critical as it will direct the choice of intervention strategies. For example, part of the data generated from an examination might include the following: a female patient has wrist pain (an impairment), is limited in the amount of typing she can do each hour (a functional limitation), and has uncharacteristically missed deadlines for data inputting in the past few weeks (a disability). If the history of the pain is one of slow onset, progressively worsening with time while typing, then one hypothesis might be that the pain is not causing the functional losses directly, but rather there is something about the task itself that is injuring. For this hypothesis, a therapist might want to address the ergonomics and work habits of the woman as the primary emphasis, with elimination of the pain as the secondary emphasis of care. If the cause of the pain were an acute sprain suffered during a weekend roller-skating accident, then the hypothesis would more likely be that the pain was directly causing limitations of typing time but that it is an injury unrelated to the nature of the typing tasks. Intervention for this hypothesis would focus on elimination of the pain as a strategy to regain functional independence, with short-term accommodation of the work environment as a secondary emphasis. In either case, linking impairments to function and patient roles through a hypothesis based on examination findings directs the clinician to choose interventions that are consistent with the hypothesized relationship.

SUMMARY

Models illustrate the relationship of concepts. They are useful for organizing information and generating hypotheses about the relationships among observations. Models of disablement illustrate the relationship between pathology and the consequences of pathology. Terminology is not consistent among models of disablement, but all address limitations of the body at the tissue level, functional limitations, and limitations in social or role participation. Some models include context or environment and personal factors. Models of disablement are useful to physical therapists for organizing patient data, guiding choices of tests and measures, diagnosing a patient problem, formulating a hypothesis about the results of an examination, and choosing intervention strategies that are consistent with the causal relationship identified in the hypothesis.

References

American Physical Therapy Association (2001). The guide to physical therapist practice. Alexandria, VA: APTA.

American Physical Therapy Association (2005). Panel describes international collaboration and standards development. PT 2005 Daily News,

June 10, from http://www.apta.org/AM/Template. cfm?Section=Search&template=/CM/HTML Display.cfm&ContentID=21891

Craik RL (1994). Disability following hip fracture. Physical Therapy 74:387–398.

Doty AK, McEwen IR, Parker D, & Laskin J (1999).

Effects of testing context on ball skill performance in 5-year-old children with and without developmental delay. Physical Therapy 79:818–826.

Haley SM, Coster WJ, & Binda-Sundberg K (1994). Measuring physical disablement: The contextual challenge. Physical Therapy 74:443–451.

Jette AM (1995). Outcomes research: Shifting the dominant research paradigm in physical therapy. Physical Therapy 75:965–970.

Jette AM (1994). Physical disablement concepts for physical therapy research and practice. Physical Therapy 74(5):380–386.

Portney LG & Watkins MP (2000). The research question. In Foundations of Clinical Research: Applications to Practice, 2nd ed., p. 122. Upper Saddle River, NJ: Prentice Hall Health.

IIISTEP Conference: Linking Movement Science and Intervention (July 15–21, 2005) at the University of Utah in Salt Lake City, Utah, organized by the Pediatric and Neurology Sections of the APTA.

US Dept. of Health and Human Services (1993). Research plan for the National Center for Medical Rehabilitation Research. NIH Pub. No. 93–3509.

Verbrugge L & Jette AM (1994). The disablement process. Social Science & Medicine 38:1–14.

World Health Organization (1980). ICIDH: International Classification of Impairments, Disabilities, and Handicaps. Geneva: World Health Organization.

World Health Organization (2001). ICF: International Classification of Functioning, Disability and Health. Geneva: World Health Organization.

EXERCISES

➤➤ Worksheet 5.1 Classification Practice

Using the ICF model of disablement, classify each of the following patient complaints as an impairment, functional limitation, or participation restriction. Identify an environmental or personal factor that would increase or reduce limitations.

Item	Classification	Factors Increasing Limitation	Factors Decreasing Limitation
Inability to button shirts			
Inability to put on shoes			
Wrist edema/ swelling			
Frequent spillage when attempting to cook			
Inability to attend religious services			
Weak grasp			

A Model of Rehabilitation Service Delivery

KEY TERMS

Inputs

Processes

Outcomes

Model

CHAPTER OUTCOMES

➤ Describe the three basic components of the Rehabilitation Service Delivery Model.

➤ Give examples of the interactions among the model components and how the components influence outcome measures.

This book approaches the study of outcomes by placing them in the context of a health services delivery model. The model is useful for organizing the variables that affect service delivery, hypothesizing relationships that might exist, and framing questions to investigate the outcomes of service delivery. The model helps the clinician identify the data to organize, the types of interventions to examine, and the types of outcomes to measure.

A MODEL OF HEALTH SERVICES DELIVERY

A simplified version of the model was first introduced by Donabedian (1966) to measure quality in health care and was adapted to explain general health services delivery (Holzemer & Reilly, 1995; Nelson, 1996). The basic components of the Health Services Delivery Model are the *inputs* and the *processes*, which combine to result in *outcomes*. Figure 6.1 illustrates the categories of the inputs, processes, and outcomes of a generic health service model.

The Inputs

Inputs are those characteristics or variables that define a particular service setting. In health service settings, the characteristics are related to the patients (or clients), the service providers, and the settings. The *patients/clients* are individuals or groups of people who receive services. They are typically described by diagnosis, age, and reason for referral. The *providers* are those people who give the services; their characteristics can include type of profession, specialized training or certification status, and years of experience. The *settings* are the places where services might be provided. Settings can be described by the level of care rendered; e.g. acute care hospitals, residential rehabilitation centers, outpatient clinics, or schools. They can also be categorized by their geographic location (e.g., country or state; demographic levels of urban, suburban, or rural), by the type of health-care system they are in (e.g., government sponsored, private, socialized), or by a type of service that is provided (e.g., general versus niche practice). In order to measure outcomes and manage practice through outcome data, it is important to record the unique characteristics of the clients, providers, and settings.

The Processes

Processes are the activities or services that patients or providers participate in. Patient processes include receipt of direct care, use of home exercise pro-

Inputs	Processes	Outcomes
Clients or patients	Client processes	Client-related outcomes
Service providers	Service processes	Service-related outcomes
Setting characteristics	Setting processes	Setting-related outcomes

Figure 6.1 Generic model of health-care systems.

grams, and participation in a support group. Provider processes include the types of examination procedures used, direct interventions delivered, and indirect interventions such as educational activities or patient advocacy with social service agencies. Setting processes include billing and scheduling procedures, documentation procedures, and continuous quality improvement processes.

The Outcomes

Outcomes are the results of the services provided relative to the service providers, the patients, and the setting characteristics. Outcomes, like inputs, can be categorized by their relevance to the patient, the provider, or the type of setting. Patient outcomes include changes in functional limitations or role participation, the cost to the patient, and patient satisfaction with the service received. Functional outcomes are changes in the client's ability to perform activities of daily living, work-related tasks, and recreational skills. Role changes include the ability to resume or adapt activities in the social networks that are important to the patient. Cost outcomes are most often considered the cost of providing services, but they can also reflect the cost of disablement to the patient, including time off from work, out-of-pocket expenses, and lost opportunity for work advancement. Patient satisfaction outcomes encompass a wide range of patient perceptions about administrative procedures, the delivery of services by the clinician, and the patient's perceptions about the results of intervention.

Provider outcomes are the results of providing services to groups of patients and relate to an individual provider or groups of providers. Examples of provider outcomes include changes in patient impairment or functional status as a result of provider interventions, frequency of success in achieving patient goals, and provider satisfaction with service provision.

Setting outcomes are the results of service provision that are meaningful to administrative levels of organizations or institutions rather than to the individual service provider. Examples of setting outcomes include the cost of providing services for a particular diagnostic group, referral rates, reimbursement patterns, and quality assurance compliance levels.

A MODEL OF REHABILITATION SERVICES DELIVERY

Figure 6.2 expands on the generic models of health service by providing specific examples of the inputs, processes, and outcomes that are relevant to rehabilitation settings; it is the model that is used throughout this book. Keep in mind that while there are many examples in each section of the model, they are not exhaustive of what might be identified. The variety of items in each section are meant to suggest what could be included in a study so that when different types of inputs, processes, or outcomes are found in the literature, they can be categorized within the structure of the model.

On the left side of Figure 6.2, *inputs* are divided into patient, provider, and setting inputs. When designing an outcome study, the clinician will need to identify which patient, provider, and/or setting characteristics are most important to include.

In the center are *processes* in which physical therapists often participate. Where possible, the language parallels the APTA Guide to Physical Therapist

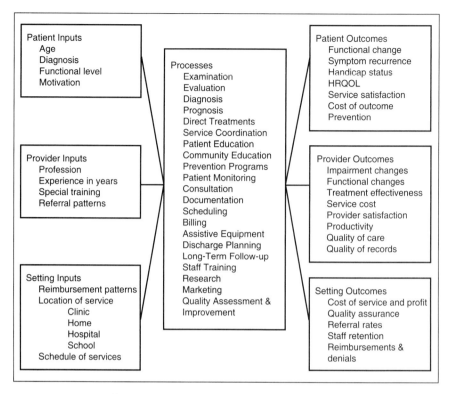

Figure 6.2 Model of Rehabilitation Service Delivery.

Practice (2001) and the ICF Model of Disablement (WHO, 2001). The list includes global descriptions of activities that need to be further defined to be useful for data collection. For example, *direct treatment* is a category of activity; the Guide to Physical Therapist Practice identifies nine domains of direct or procedural intervention, such as therapeutic exercise, functional training, and manual therapy (APTA, 2001, p. 106), and these activities can be further defined into types of interventions or protocols (Box 6.1).

On the right are the *outcomes,* divided into patient, provider, and setting outcomes. The language of disablement models is apparent within the patient

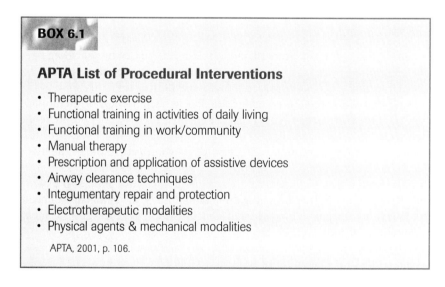

and provider outcome sections. In the patient outcomes, these categories are important to the patient as personal markers of change. In the provider section, they are relevant to the provider as more generic measures of intervention or therapist effectiveness.

There are some outcomes that have not been typically reported in physical therapy literature but are increasingly included in health services studies; these include health-related quality of life (HRQOL), cost of outcome to the patient, and provider satisfaction. Certain provider and setting outcomes, such as provider productivity, cost of service, referral rates, and measures of staff retention, have typically been perceived as internal management measures to support administrative decisions, development of clinical pathways, and even merit awards. Many of these administrative measures are becoming more public as health service providers compete with each other for greater shares of the market. However, regardless of why they may be more or less prevalent in the literature, the emphasis on cost-effective service delivery will facilitate studies of intervention effectiveness and HRQOL.

The expanded Model of Rehabilitation Service Delivery is useful for illustrating the complexity of health service delivery. A single patient outcome is often the result of more than just a single input or intervention. As stated in Chapter 2, all outcomes are relative to the interaction of the inputs, processes, and outcome measures that were used during an episode of care.

At the beginning of a study, the clinician should use the model to identify the characteristics that may influence a single outcome. After data are collected, the clinician should use the model to appreciate the characteristics and variables that were *not* included in the data set; those variables need to be recognized for their potential impact on the results.

THE INTERACTION OF INPUTS AND PROCESSES RESULTING IN OUTCOMES

The lines that connect the different portions of the Model of Rehabilitation Service Delivery represent the hypothetical relationships among the three major categories. Any combination of characteristics can be studied; the choice of characteristics will depend on the question being asked. Look at the following examples of relationships based on the model.

Simple Designs

In Figure 6.3 there are three examples of relationships that might be studied. In the first example, changes in patient satisfaction would be measured before and after a new scheduling procedure is put into effect. The scheduling procedure may have been created to address a particular need of evening patients, and so only evening patients are included in the data set. A patient satisfaction survey that yields some overall score is used to measure the impact of the new procedure.

In the second example, a clinician is interested in whether patients with strokes change some aspect of their functional status after receiving interventions.

In the third example, a clinician is interested in what effect a pain management program has on HRQOL scores for patients with chronic low back pain. Both immediate and long-term effects of the education program could be measured by administering a standardized HRQOL survey to patients

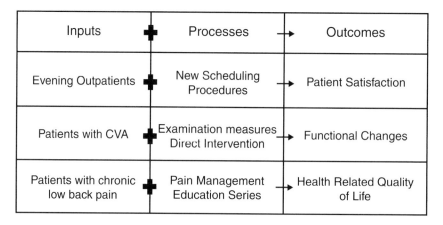

Figure 6.3 Examples of simple study designs organized by the model.

before the first class, 1 month after the last class, and then 4 months after the last class. This type of data would be most helpful in understanding the enduring benefits of an educational intervention.

All three examples have broadly identified a type of input, process, and outcome to illustrate possible relationships. If studies were actually carried out to explore any of the examples, additional clarification of terms would be needed.

What is most important to realize from these examples is that changes in outcome measures are directly associated with the service delivery environment from which they are derived. In Figure 6.3 the scheduling procedure, the types of interventions that patients with cardiovascular accidents (CVAs) receive, and the actual curriculum of a chronic pain management program are unique to those settings and talents of the clinicians who carry them out. The same scheduling procedure (*process*) might be very effective in one setting and ineffective in another because of the type of patients (*inputs*) or the preferences of the providers. Evaluating the relationship between examinations and interventions (*process*) and functional outcomes (*outcome*) is useful for predicting change, but the strength of any association is a function of the unique setting (*input*) in which services are rendered. The severity of the patients' conditions (*input*) and the theoretical models that the clinicians use to administer direct care (*process*) are just two variables that can affect results even in the same clinical setting. Likewise, a pain management curriculum taught in one setting using an interactive discussion approach (*process*) might yield vastly different results than if taught in the same setting using a straight lecture format (*process*).

Complex Designs

The relationships illustrated in Figure 6.3 are somewhat simple in design and may be the appropriate level of complexity for a pilot study. As the clinician begins to explore simpler relationships in the data, other variables may be identified that influence the outcome measure.

Figure 6.4 illustrates a more complex relationship of interactions to demonstrate how the design can be used for more complex questions. There are three types of inputs described: the patients with CVAs, the physician referral patterns, and the type of health-care benefits that each patient

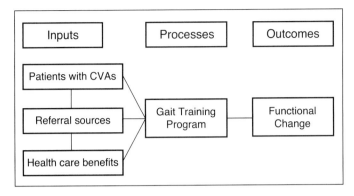

Figure 6.4 Example of increasing study complexity using the model.

has. Identifying selected characteristics of each type of input allows for a more detailed picture of each patient. Subsets of patients can then be made by grouping patients with the same referral source and type of insurance plan.

Figure 6.5 illustrates how these subsets might look. By dividing the patient sample according to the side of lesion, referral sources by those who

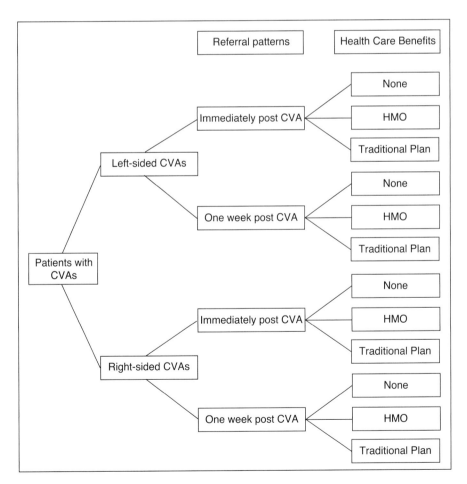

Figure 6.5 Example of a complex study resulting in 12 subsets of patient groups.

refer immediately and those who wait 1 week, and the benefits category by 3 types of payment options, 12 subsets of patient groups are created. Each subset is described by the referral source and type of health-care benefit, and the outcome data are the scores on the functional examinations for each patient in a subset. Clearly, as more variables are included, more subsets are formed, and more patients need to be included to have adequate data representation in each subset.

There are numerous variations that could have been proposed in Figure 6.5. At first glance, it might seem obvious that a more complex design would be more useful for predicting outcomes and planning interventions, but that can be answered only by the person asking the initial question. It might be possible to simplify the design by omitting a characteristic in any one of the categories. For example, if the interest were specifically about those patients with left-sided CVAs, only the top half of the design would need to be studied, and that would reduce the number of subsets to six. Alternately, if a clinic served very few people with traditional forms of health insurance plans, then that characteristic could be omitted, and that would result in eight subsets of patients. In either case, reducing the number of subsets may answer a question more directly, reduce the time it takes to collect and enter data, and may simplify the statistical work that is needed to provide an answer to the question.

SUMMARY

The Model of Rehabilitation Service Delivery is presented as a tool to help organize the question for an outcome study, to assist in identifying the variables that might influence the outcome results, and to help the clinician interpret the results of a study by framing the variables that are studied against those that are not. Each clinician must appreciate the uniqueness of the clinical setting in which services are delivered and how outcome measures are reflections of a dynamic interaction of multiple inputs and processes. Using the Model of Rehabilitation Service Delivery requires each clinician to hypothesize which inputs and processes are uniquely associated with the desired outcome measures. Developing the hypothesized relationships and clearly describing the characteristics of interest *before* data are collected will save the clinician time during the data collection phase and keep the data set simple but useful.

References

American Physical Therapy Association (2001). The guide to physical therapist practice, 2nd edition. Physical Therapy 81:1–798.

Camp PG, Appleton J, & Reid WD (2000). Quality of life after pulmonary rehabilitation: Assessing change using quantitative and qualitative methods. Physical Therapy 80:986–995.

Donabedian A. (1966). Evaluating the quality of medical care. Milbank Quarterly 44: 166–206.

Geiger RA, Allen JB, O'Keefe J, & Hicks RR (2001). Balance and mobility following stroke: Effects of physical therapy interventions with and without biofeedback/forceplate training. Physical Therapy 81:995–1005.

Holzemer WL & Reilly CA (1995). Variables, variability, and variations research: Implications for medial informatics. Journal of the American Medical Informatics Association 2:183–190.

Ketelaar M, Vermeer A, 't Hart H, van Petegem-van Beek E, & Helders PJM (2001). Effects of a functional therapy program on motor abilities of children with cerebral palsy. Physical Therapy 81:1534–1545.

Nelson MK (1996). Measuring the cost of health care services: An accounting perspective.

Presented at APTA Workshop "Collecting and using patient data: an interactive workshop on outcome measures." Chicago.

World Health Organization (2001). ICF: International Classification of Functioning, Disability and Health. Geneva: World Health Organization.

EXERCISES

Use the Model of Rehabilitation Service Delivery to dissect the relationships tested by the following studies.

Example 1. <u>Purpose of the Study</u>: "to examine whether the motor abilities of children with cerebral palsy who were receiving functional physical therapy improved more than the motor abilities of children in a reference group whose therapy was based on the principle of normalization of the quality of movement." Ketelaar, et al. (2001), p. 1537.

<u>Inputs:</u>

<u>Processes:</u>

<u>Outputs:</u>

Example 2. <u>Purpose of the Study</u>: "to compare outcomes (using the Berg Balance Scale and the Timed Up & Go Test) following balance and mobility retraining by physical therapy with and without the addition of NeuroCom Balance Master training in 2 groups of patients who had hemiplegia secondary to stroke." Geiger, et al. (2001), p. 997.

<u>Inputs:</u>

<u>Processes:</u>

<u>Outputs:</u>

Example 3. <u>Purpose of the Study</u>: "to determine the changes in QOL (quality of life) in individuals with COPD (Chronic Obstructive Pulmonary Disease) who have undergone a pulmonary rehabilitation program using both quantitative and qualitative research methods." Camp, et al. (2000), p. 988.

<u>Inputs:</u>

<u>Processes:</u>

<u>Outputs:</u>

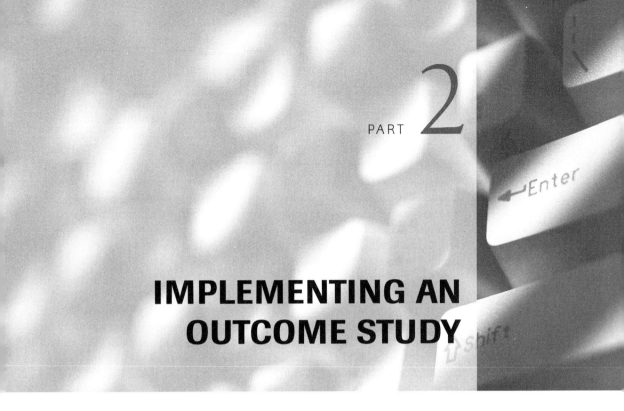

PART 2

IMPLEMENTING AN OUTCOME STUDY

PART 2
IMPLEMENTING AN OUTCOME STUDY

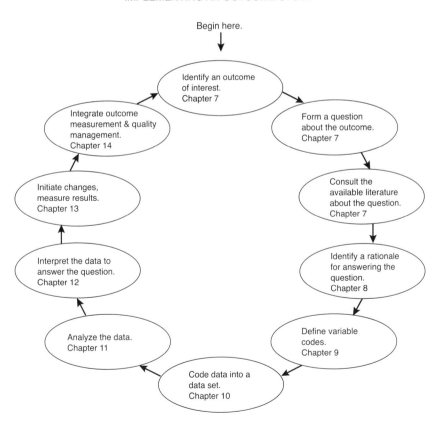

Begin here.

Identify an outcome
of interest.
Chapter 7

Form a question
about the outcome.
Chapter 7

Consult the
available literature
about the question.
Chapter 7

Identify a rationale
for answering the
question.
Chapter 8

Define variable
codes.
Chapter 9

Code data into a
data set.
Chapter 10

Analyze the data.
Chapter 11

Interpret the data to
answer the question.
Chapter 12

Initiate changes,
measure results.
Chapter 13

Integrate outcome
measurement & quality
management.
Chapter 14

Introduction: Implementing an Outcome Study

The process of measuring outcomes is a circular process that starts with the identification of a problem. The figure illustrates the major steps in the process, and the chapters in this section follow the order of these steps. In Chapters 7 and 8, the steps of evidence-based practice are merged with the processes of outcome measurement. The parallels are very strong and may provide a more familiar approach for identifying an answerable question. Chapters 9, 10, and 11 describe the processes of data coding, organization, and analysis. Chapter 12 provides strategies for writing a report of the outcome results, with emphasis on how to tailor reports for different audiences.

Because objective and consistent documentation processes are at the heart of outcome measurement, a study of documentation patterns is provided at the end of this section to illustrate each step. This type of study is recommended as a first step for readers who are embarking on outcome studies for the first time. In Appendix 1, the steps of a pilot study on documentation patterns is provided for readers to complete, using data from their own clinical practice setting. Conducting this study of documentation will help to identify the strengths and limitations of the clinician's available data; this is an essential step before embarking on clinical outcome studies. A mock data set has been provided in Appendix 3 for those who do not have access to patient records.

The focus of this book is on teaching the steps of outcome measurement as the basis for improving the services of the individual clinician. Consequently, it is recommended that the first attempts at outcome measurement be limited to records of patients treated by the clinician reader. If the clinician uses physical therapy records of patients he or she personally managed from start to finish, then assembling a data set for self-reflection should not require institutional approval nor will the clinician be violating any confidentialities as he or she wrote the notes. However, if the clinician intends to publish the results of a study or use records of patients treated by other therapists, the clinician must seek approval from the clinic's institutional review board for permission to use confidential records. In any case, the investigating clinician should refer to his/her own institution's policies and procedures for retrospective chart review.

Developing a Question

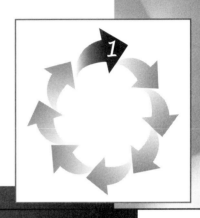

KEY TERMS

Answerable question

PICO

PIO

Model of Rehabilitation Service
 Delivery

Evidence-based practice

Literature search

Internet resources

Data mining

CHAPTER OUTCOMES

➤ Develop an answerable question for an out-come study.

➤ Use the Model of Rehabilitation Service Delivery to illustrate hypothesized rela-tionships among inputs, processes, and outcomes.

➤ Describe strategies for searching the literature and other information sources.

Performing outcome measurement begins with identifying a meaningful and answerable question. Once the question has been determined, the inputs and processes related to the outcome of interest are identified. In this chapter, the origins of outcome questions are described, and sample questions about clinical practice are organized using the Model of Rehabilitation Service Delivery and evidence-based practice strategies.

IDENTIFY AN OUTCOME OF INTEREST

The first step in any outcome study is to identify the outcome of interest. The choice might be based on interesting clinical observations, an issue raised in the literature, a question from someone about an aspect of practice, or a management concern. It is more meaningful to study an aspect of practice that is important or pressing. The process of outcome measurement requires a long-term commitment, so the chosen question and outcome should hold the clinician's interest over time, and the answer should be useful in practice.

In some way, the chosen outcome should be related to improving patient services. Whether at the level of the individual patient or at broader level of service delivery to many patients, the purpose of outcome measurement is to influence service provision. This focus on improving services is one of the key differences between outcome research and other types of research. In basic science, or "bench," research, discovery for the sake of identifying a new entity or relationship is purpose enough. In contrast, outcome research is conducted specifically to improve the quality of services provided. If a link between the question, the possible answers, and managerial or clinical strategies is not clear, then the question may not be suitable for an outcome study.

➤ *Outcome research is conducted to improve the quality of service delivery.*

Outcome studies have different origination points. A study might begin with a request from a hospital administrator to determine patient satisfaction with services in a clinical setting. In this example, the starting point is at the *outcome* portion of the model; that is, patient satisfaction is a type of *patient outcome*. The *inputs* in this study might include all outpatients served during a particular month, and the *process* might be limited to patients who received only direct services, but the inputs and processes are determined after the outcome is identified.

An outcome study can examine a *process*. Suppose a manager wanted to review the quality of *documentation* in a clinical setting. In this type of a study, the input characteristics and outcome measures will help to define the sample size of the medical records that will need to be reviewed. This study of documentation could select patients with a particular diagnosis of patella-femoral knee pain *(patient inputs)* and who received a particular service, such as physical therapy *(the process)*. The *outcome* might be to determine how many records had complete documentation. The criteria for "complete documentation" would need to be defined operationally, and then all the medical records would be categorized against these criteria. The question might look like: "What percentage of patient records meets the internal quality assurance standards *(outcome)* for documentation *(process of interest)* for patients treated for patella-femoral knee pain *(patient input)* by this physical therapy department *(setting input)*?"

Finally, a study can begin with an interest in a particular patient group. If a clinician has many patients with a particular type of injury or has patients with a diagnosis that seems to have variable results, it may clarify practice patterns to review their charts objectively. Coding the presenting symptoms of the patients, what services the patients received, and patient outcomes can shed light on the patterns of services provided and actual versus perceived clinical effectiveness of the clinician.

CREATING AN ANSWERABLE QUESTION

Once an issue or question is identified, it needs to be framed so it can be answered. The process of honing a question to accurately reflect the issue is important because broad questions yield broad answers; they are difficult to apply to specific clinical decisions. Because the purpose of outcome measurement is to improve the clinician's effectiveness with patients, the question needs to address the individual clinician's concerns accurately.

➤ *General questions = general answers*

Suppose a clinician is interested in describing patients with multiple sclerosis (MS) after they have been treated in the clinician's practice setting. The starting point is the interest in a patient sample, a type of *patient input*. Specifically, the clinician might be interested in the patients' change in functional status (*outcome*) when discharged from services. The initial question might be: "What is the functional status of my patients with MS at discharge from my services?"

Although this is an interesting question, it may not be easy to answer because it is very broad. The patient sample is inclusive of many characteristics, and functional status is inclusive of many types of activities. For this question, the discharge level of functional status might depend on the level of symptom severity or the time since onset of symptoms. Additionally, it could depend on the amount of intervention a patient receives or the types of intervention provided. As there are so many variables, it would be helpful to focus on the particular patients with MS for whom the clinician most needs answers. The scope of the question can be narrowed using either the Model of Rehabilitation Service Delivery or the steps of evidence-based practice.

Model of Rehabilitation Service Delivery

To use the Model of Rehabilitation Service Delivery, place the variables in the question into the appropriate components of the model (Fig. 7.1).

Inputs

Other than identifying the diagnosis of interest, there are no other patient inputs in this version of the question, such as age, gender, or date of onset of the diagnosis. There are no characteristics of the providers or the setting, and there are no processes identified. To answer this broad question, all patients with multiple sclerosis who have been treated by this clinician and who received any type of service would need to be included in the sample. The answer will be very broad because it will include a wide variety of patients with MS who received services for many different functional limitations. (This is like mixing many varieties of apples and trying to say something about their contribution to applesauce.) To improve the usefulness of the answer to this question, the inputs, processes, and outcomes need to be further defined.

If more patient characteristics are included, the eligibility criteria for the sample become more selective, which allows the answer to be applied to a

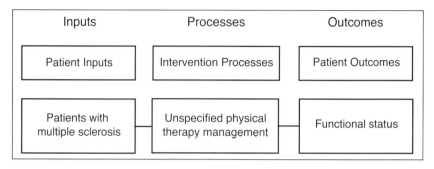

Figure 7.1 Initial question with variables placed in the model of rehabilitation services.

more specific group of patients. Depending on the interest of the clinician, the patient inputs can be narrowed by time of onset (e.g., patients diagnosed in the past 4 months), by a cluster of symptoms (e.g., patients with vertigo), by age (e.g., patients 30–50 years old), or by some combination of characteristics. Similar groups of patients can be studied, such as those who receive different interventions, or groups with different clusters of symptoms to understand the symptoms' impact on functional outcomes. The point is that if the type of patient problem can be narrowed to describe a specific cluster of characteristics, the answer to the question will be more useful in clinical decision making.

➤ *Specific questions = specific answers*

In addition to patient inputs, provider and setting inputs should be identified. Provider inputs include the types of service, the experience of the providers, and the approaches that providers use. The setting inputs can be identified by location (e.g., urban, suburban, and rural), type of health-care service (e.g., socialized versus private), type of payment source (e.g., private pay, third party payment), or type of environment (e.g., hospital, skilled nursing facility, wellness center, or elementary school). Even characteristics of settings, such as the average time spent individually with patients or access that people have to services (e.g., a corporate on-site clinic, direct access, or access by precertification) can influence the outcomes. Thus, defining the unique characteristics of the *providers* and *service settings* are equally important.

Processes

The next part of the model and question to focus on are the *processes* or *interventions*. Accurate descriptions of the processes or interventions clarify what happens to the patient as well as what is *not* included or accounted for in a study. When the results are interpreted, there may be processes that influence the outcomes for which the study did not or could not account, and the clinician needs to recognize these. Examples might include the use of a standardized test applied at admission and at discharge or the provision of a type of intervention. The narrowed question might now read, "What are the functional outcomes for patients with MS who use assistive devices to walk, who were treated in a suburban outpatient clinic by this physical therapist who has certification as a neurological specialist, and who exercise with or without a cooling vest?"

In this revised question, the patient inputs are defined by the diagnosis (MS) and a level of functioning (use of assistive devices to walk). The provider inputs are described in part by the discipline and the professional

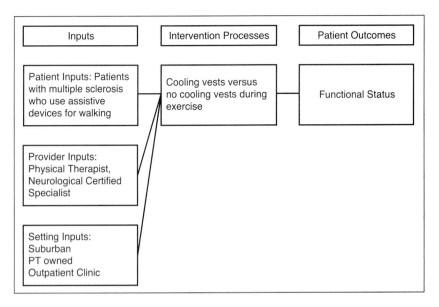

Figure 7.2 Sample question with greater detail in the model of rehabilitation services.

certification. The setting inputs are described by locale and type of service setting. The processes are further defined as exercise with or without a cooling vest. When reframed in the Model of Rehabilitation Service Delivery, the question would look as depicted in Figure 7.2.

Outcome

Now the people and the processes are more specific, but the functional outcome is not defined well. Functional outcomes can be described by any number of activities and tasks that a person performs. The clinician needs to identify exactly what should improve as a result of the intervention. Consider this list of possible functional outcomes:

- Improved score on a 6-minute walk test
- Faster walking speed with or without assistive devices
- Number of patients who can shed or reduce the size of their current assistive device
- Improved ability to walk over varied surfaces with or without assistive devices
- Improved tolerance for exercise as measured by time

Any of these, and many more, can serve as an operational definition for the *functional outcome;* it all depends on what the clinician is interested in. If one outcome is picked and placed in the question, it will read as follows: "What are the changes in the 6-minute walk test for patients with MS who use assistive devices to walk, who were treated in a suburban outpatient clinic by this physical therapist who has certification as a neurological specialist, and who exercise with or without a cooling vest?"

Placing the question in the Model of Rehabilitation Service Delivery further clarifies the relationships of the inputs to processes and outcome. When the initial question (see Fig. 7.1) is compared with the current form of the question (Fig. 7.3), the process of narrowing the scope of the question by

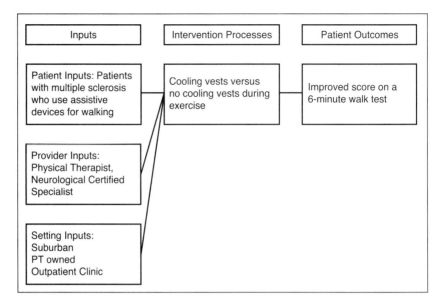

Figure 7.3 Further refinement of the question.

using the model is evident. The first question is broad and could generate any number of answers depending on who the patients are, what interventions they receive, and what is defined as the outcome. The third version of the question is more focused, and the answer to this question will be more easily related to practice because the inputs, processes, and outputs are more focused.

What should also be appreciated are all of the variables that are *not* addressed in this simplified example. This is easy to see when the question is superimposed on the Model of Rehabilitation Service Delivery, as in Figure 7-4. The model has many more variables identified as examples of inputs and processes, among which are the variables from the sample question. Many of the inputs and processes that are not addressed in this question might influence the outcome. The clinician will need to determine those critical variables on which to collect data and those variables that are "nice to know" but not necessary for the study. In addition, when it is time to analyze and interpret the data, the clinician may find it useful to refer to the model as a reminder of what was *not* included or controlled for in the data collection. This will help the clinician avoid a common pitfall of overgeneralizing results, without regard for other variables that might confound the results.

Converting the Question Into a PICO or PIO Format

The PICO or PIO format is a question format that provides another method for converting a broad question into an answerable question. The acronym provides a structure for the investigator to relate the characteristics of the patient sample and the process of interest to a measurable outcome.

The structure of a PICO or PIO question is borrowed from the literature on evidence-based practice (cebm.net/focus_quest.asp). The acronym represents the parts of an answerable question.

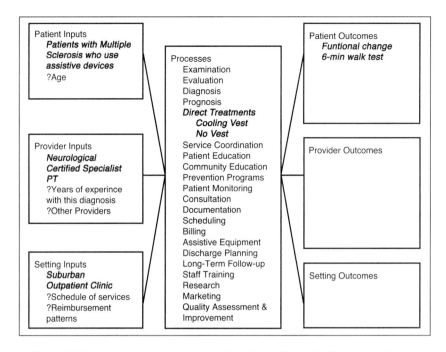

Figure 7.4 Superimposing the question onto the Model of Rehabilitation Service Delivery.

P is the patient, patient group, or problem of interest.

I is any intervening activity provided to the patient, group, or problem.

C is an optional comparison intervention or activity.

O is the outcome of interest expressed as a measurable quality.

The PICO format parallels the Model of Rehabilitation Service Delivery as follows:

P is the patient, provider, and service setting inputs.

I is one of the processes of interest.

C is a comparison process.

O is the outcome of interest expressed as a measurable quality.

Framing a question using this acronym helps to identify the key inputs, processes, and outcomes of interest. The P should identify as much about the patient as might be relevant, e.g., age, diagnosis with severity level if appropriate, type of environment, and types of support. The P should include all of the relevant *inputs* identified in the Model of Rehabilitation Service Delivery.

The I is broader than the traditional physical therapy interpretation of the term "intervention," which is often equated with treatment. The I refers to any activity, including examination techniques, direct patient treatments, educational interventions, alterations in equipment, or changes in marketing approaches. The I is equated with the *processes* in the Model of Rehabilitation Service Delivery. If two interventions are being compared, the question will have all four parts of the PICO structure, with C as a comparison intervention. If the question is exploratory or descriptive in nature, or if a comparison intervention or activity is not appropriate, then the question will have only three parts, resulting in a PIO format, without a C comparison.

The O needs to result in a number. It is not acceptable to use an up ($\uparrow$) or down ($\downarrow$) arrow or terms like "improved" in the outcome statement, because it is not possible to determine objectively if a meaningful change in the outcome has occurred. Thus, all outcome statements should identify a score, a measurement, or some quantifiable characteristic such as speed or time that can be recorded.

A simple study may have a single outcome measure, resulting in a traditional PICO format. Descriptive studies may have several outcomes, or Os. In this case, the question format will look like PIOO or PICOOO, with one O for each outcome of interest. This format is especially useful when the clinician is exploring a variety of outcomes that are hypothesized to be related to selected inputs and processes.

Here are some sample questions presented in PICO or PIO formats.

Example 1

P   For my patients with MS who use assistive devices to walk, who are treated in a suburban outpatient clinic

I   who exercised for 1 hour with a cooling vest

C   compared with those who did not use a cooling vest

O   what are their changes in the 6-minute walk test after 4 weeks of intervention?

Example 2

P   For outpatients in my clinic

I   who received direct services during a particular month

O   what is the level of patient satisfaction?

Example 3

P   For patients with a diagnosis of patella-femoral knee pain, with medical records

I   that meet out internal documentation criteria

C   as compared with those records with documentation deficiencies

O   what is the percentage of charts that meet criteria?

O   does one group have a higher success rate of reimbursement?

USING AVAILABLE DATA TO DEVELOP A QUESTION

There is one more way that outcome studies can originate, and that is from existing data sets. Every clinical setting generates a wealth of data on which outcome studies can be performed. Some of those data are collected routinely but used only for billing or census support. Depending on the setting, some of the data may be collected by separate departments, such as a registration department, a rehabilitation department, or a laboratory or medical clinic. Typical electronic medical records include the patient's demographic information, reason for referral, diagnostic codes, and intervention codes. Those data can be useful for understanding management processes, service utilization, and patient outcomes.

The key to using these data is having access to data sets. Large data sets may be available after having been cleaned of identifying information, or they can be created from other data sets that are being managed for other purposes (such as billing software). If the facility has an information management or bioinformatics department, that department may be able to create a subset of the filtered data to study.

This process of sifting through large sets of data to identify trends and relationships within the data is called *data mining* (Edelstein, 2004). Whole textbooks are written to teach the skills and techniques to mine very large databases, but the concept and approach is introduced here as an alternative source of study for the reflective clinician.

When data sets are available, the process of developing a question is somewhat reversed. First, the data are reviewed to see what types of variables are included. Questions are developed based on the available data. The intent is to explore relationships among the variables in order to create a *prediction model* based on known results or to create a *descriptive pattern* to guide future decisions. In the case of outcome measurement, either is possible, but describing patterns to guide future decisions is more consistent with retrospective studies. Thus, existing data are reviewed, and trends in current service delivery are described to objectively validate assumptions about service delivery or to answer questions about service utilization.

Regardless of whether a question is derived from clinical curiosity about patient inputs or from the need to describe specific outcomes or as a result of mining an existing data set, the next step in the process is reviewing the related literature.

GOING TO THE LITERATURE

Why Go to the Literature?

After the question is clarified, a thorough review of related literature is conducted to see if the question has already been answered, to see how it has (or has not) been studied, and to identify what is already known about the question. All the inputs and processes should be reviewed to understand their role in the study and how they are the same or different from those in related studies. The outcome measures should be reviewed for established validity and reliability as well as for methods of measurement. This information will determine whether to proceed with the chosen outcome measures, and it will influence how the results are interpreted.

If there is literature specifically answering the same question that has been posed (a rare find indeed), it is important to identify whether the clinician's practice setting is similar to the setting in the published study. Many studies are conducted in controlled laboratory environments in which prospective patient samples are controlled for similarity, or interventions are controlled to be consistent across all participants. The laboratory environment is not like the clinical environment. In the clinic, patients are treated as they arrive, receive treatment tailored to their individual needs, and sample groups for outcome studies are constructed through retrospective chart sampling. Thus, even if articles related directly to the question are found, the results may still need to be interpreted with caution for their direct application in a clinical practice environment.

Where to Search

There are many sources that should be checked for studies that have previously answered the question. Access through electronic databases of publications has made the searching process more time-efficient. Internet access allows anyone to peruse national library holdings through Pub Med (ncbi. nlm.nih.gov/entrez/query.fcgi) and online journal collections such as freemedicaljournals.com. Librarians are available in medical centers and public libraries to assist the novice with conducting complete searches. Several excellent sources on searching for literature and critical appraisal of literature are provided in the list of recommended readings at the end of this chapter.

WHAT IF NO LITERATURE IS FOUND?

Students and clinicians are often surprised to find that few or no studies exist to answer their exact question. Quite often, the first response is to try to change the question to match the literature that is available. Resist that inclination! If the question has been carefully identified so that the answer will improve clinical decision making or help inform patient care plans, then stay true to your rationale, and continue to attempt to answer the question. Here are some suggestions for how to proceed.

1. **Review the search terms**. Be sure to use single search terms, synonyms, and related terminology. Try British spellings, generic categories, and related concepts.
2. **Search a variety of sources**. Most clinicians are familiar with Medline (Pub Med) and the National Library of Medicine, but there are many other sources that should be queried. Other relevant journal databases include the Cumulative Index of Nursing and Allied Health Literature (cinahl.com/); PsycINFO, which has psychology literature (apa.org/psycinfo/); and ERIC, which has education literature (eric.ed.gov/). The National Guideline Clearinghouse (guideline.gov/) contains medical guidelines posted according to set criteria, and the Cochrane Collaboration (cochrane.org/index0.htm) is a database of evidence-based systematic reviews. CATs are Critically Appraised Topics, and CAT Banks or databases of CATs or BETs (Best Evidence Topics) are on the increase. A visit to the Centre for Evidence-Based Medicine's website (cebm.net/index.asp) provides information about CATs and links to existing CAT banks.
3. **Search all health-care professions**. Physical therapists like to see what other physical therapists have studied, but limiting a search to "physical therapy" may eliminate important studies from nursing or medicine that could shed light on the question.
4. **Avoid common search mistakes**. Do not limit the search to "full text" options so that the article can be downloaded immediately; many articles will be missed that way. Look at widest available collection of citations, and narrow them down by reading the abstracts. Then collect the articles, whether by full text downloads from online sources or by finding the journals in a library collection. Search multiple databases as not all peer-reviewed journals qualify for listing on Medline. Do not be afraid to go back in time; just because an article is 10 or 20 or more years old does not mean it may not be useful. Sometimes the original studies reveal theoretical assumptions that may play key roles in the application or interpretation of data or in clinical decision making.
5. **Study individual characteristics.** If combined search terms are initially entered to represent the inputs, the processes, and the outcomes, and nothing is found, then consider searching each part separately. The search may turn up studies of similar patients with the same functional assessment but having a different intervention. It may find studies of patients with similar diagnoses who received the same intervention but who have different outcome measures. From these studies, the clinician will need to piece together a framework of related findings that help to predict the outcomes of the clinician's sample. These peripherally related studies shed light

on operational definitions, measurement techniques, and data analysis approaches taken by others who have studied similar patients, interventions, or outcomes.

6. **Visit the websites of related organizations.** Many nonprofit and patient advocacy organizations keep track of literature related to the diagnostic group they represent. Organizations such as the American Heart Association and United Cerebral Palsy maintain resource sites on their web pages as well as provide links to other sites. In solving clinical questions, the best available evidence can come from many resources, not only journal articles, and in the absence of any journal articles, expert opinion or consensus statements may be useful for understanding the context of an outcome question.

7. **Shift the focus from answers to theory.** When the question has not been directly studied in the literature, it may be necessary to step back from the desire for a factual answer and to identify the theoretical foundations that might guide the development of other potential answers.

After completing the literature and resource searches, print out the history of the searches to keep track of the strategies used. After data collection and analysis are completed, it is appropriate to conduct another search of the literature to see if anything has been published since the initial search.

SUMMARY

Outcome studies begin with asking a question about some aspect of service delivery in which the clinician is interested. That question may come from clinical experiences, a desire to improve service delivery, or an issue that arises in the literature or from mining an existing data set. The process of questioning begins in any section of the Model of Rehabilitation Service Delivery. Regardless of its starting point, the outcome question should specify the inputs, processes, and outcome measurements that are unique to the clinician's service delivery patterns so that the answer is useful in practice. Once the question is clarified, the literature and other sources should be reviewed to see if the question has been answered before or to see what new knowledge is available about the variables in the question.

References

Centre for Evidence-Based Medicine (2003). Focusing Clinical Questions. (www.cebm.net/focus_quest.asp)

Edelstein, H (2004). Mining large databases: A case study. Two Crows Corporation. twocrows.com/articles.htm

Recommended Resources

Evidence-Based Practice

Law M (ed). (2002). Evidence-based rehabilitation; A guide to practice. Slack Inc, Thorofare, NJ.

Sackett DL, et al. (2000). Evidence-Based Medicine:

How to Practice and Teach EBM. Churchill Livingstone, NY.

Searching For and Organizing the Literature

Garrard J (1999). Health Sciences Literature Review Made Easy: The Matrix Method. Aspen Publishers, Inc. Gaithersburg, MD.

Websites

Agency for Healthcare Research and Quality (ahrq.gov)

BETs - Best Evidence Topics (bestbets.org/index.html)

CATs - Critically Appraised Topics (urmc.rochester.edu/MEDICINE/RES/CATS/index.html)

Centre for Evidence-Based Medicine (cebm.net/index.asp)

Cochrane Collaboration (cochrane.org)

National Guideline Clearinghouse (guideline.gov)

EXERCISES

Place the following questions into the Model for Rehabilitation Service Delivery.

1. What are the levels of patient satisfaction following 2 and 4 weeks of intervention by patients with acute plantar fasciitis?

2. What interventions are utilized by early intervention therapists for infants with torticollis during the first 3 weeks of home visits?

Identify the problems with the following PICO and PIO questions:

3. P: For children with cerebral palsy
   I: does stretching at home
   C: or strengthening at home
   O: improve gait and balance?

4. P: For adults with rotator cuff injuries
   I: does a change of 2 points on a visual analogue scale
   C: compared with a 4 point change
   O: result in easier overhead reaching?

5. P: How does the pain level change for my patients
   I: who receive ultrasound
   O: for 2 weeks of treatment?

Identifying a Rationale for the Study

KEY TERMS

Rationale

Action plans

Descriptive studies

Comparative studies

CHAPTER OUTCOMES

➤ Describe the benefits of identifying a rationale for conducting an outcome study.

➤ Identify four reasons for conducting outcome studies.

After the outcome question is refined and the pertinent literature is reviewed, but before the data collection process is designed, it is important to identify the *rationale* for conducting the study. The clinician should be clear about why the study should be conducted and how the results of the investigation will be used in practice. Outcome studies, even when limited to one clinician's patient care practice, require an investment of time and energy. This chapter will describe the reasons for identifying a rationale and how to integrate it with the outcome question.

THE RATIONALE: AN OPERATIONAL DEFINITION

The rationale explains the purpose for conducting the study. The rationale includes a hypothesis about the relationship among the selected inputs, processes, and outcomes and how the potential results will be applied in practice. (See Fig. 8-1 for an example of a rationale.) Regardless of whether the rationale is based on theory or practical factors, it should provide an explanation for the choice of characteristics and interventions to study as well as describe how the study results will improve service delivery.

P - For a random selection of patients discharged during the past month from this hospital outpatient facility

I - for whom this clinician wrote the goals of care,

O - what is the distribution of impairment goals?

O - what is the distribution of functional limitation goals?

O - and what is the distribution of social/role goals?

Rationale for the Sample Question.

Patient satisfaction data in this department indicates that patients do not always understand their goals. Management would like to see improvement in this area. It was hypothesized that patients don't understand their goals because the goals focus on changes in impairments rather than functional activities. Management will evaluate the frequency with which goals focus on changing impairments, functional limitations or social limitations.

Predicted use of the data:

If there is a bias toward impairment goals:
      Therapists will receive education on writing functionally oriented goals.
      Measurement of goal frequencies will reoccur in 2 months.

If the emphasis is already on function:
      The measurability of the goals will be investigated.
      Measurement of functional goal measurability will reoccur in 2 months.

If the emphasis is on social limitations, literature reviews will be conducted to:
      Determine the relationship of functional measures to social measures.
      Identify objective measures of social/role limitations.

Figure 8.1 Example of an outcome question, a rationale, and the predicted use of data.

Why a Rationale Is Needed

Outcome studies should not be started unless the clinician can answer the question, "How will the results be used?" The rationale puts the study in perspective and guides the clinician in the use of the results.

There are three possible results for most *comparative* outcome studies. The results may show that

- "Variable A" is better than "Variable B"
- "Variable B" is better than "Variable A"
- "Variable A" is equivalent to "Variable B"

In *descriptive* studies, in which the clinician identifies the incidence of a particular variable or process, there are four possible answers. The data may show

- Strong evidence for the variable or process
- Strong evidence against the variable or process
- The variable or process appears equivalent to other variables or processes
- No support for the variable or process

In a well-considered rationale, there is a plan of action for **each** of the possible outcomes. Thus, in a comparison study, if variable A appears better than variable B, the clinician might plan to use A more often. If B appears better than A, then the opposite might occur. If there is no difference between A and B, the clinician might choose randomly between them, or use the one that is more comfortable, or look for something more effective than both of them. In all cases, the clinician should plan additional follow-up measures for whatever action is taken.

The clinician should not worry about being locked into using the predicted plans based on the hypothetical results of the study. The predicted plans can and should change based on the actual results. *Predicting a plan of action* will keep the study focused and improve the likelihood that only essential data are being collected and analyzed.

Having a clear understanding of why a study is undertaken and how it will influence the delivery of rehabilitation services is helpful in focusing the time, expense, and effort invested. The goal is to conduct a study as efficiently as possible. The truth is that all investigations, no matter what size they are or how they are designed, suffer from Murphy's Law. Some things will go wrong unexpectedly and require additional time, expense, and effort. When these most frustrating moments occur, a clear rationale reinforces the commitment to the process and helps the clinician through these challenges.

> ➤ *Do not start a study without knowing how an answer will influence clinical practice.*

> ➤ *Have an action plan for each possible outcome and a plan to measure again after implementation.*

The Rationale Should Be Specific

The rationale for conducting a study should be specific to the clinician's practice setting and environment. The rationale should clearly link the variables and outcomes with the proposed action plans. Delineating the specific variables and outcomes unique to the clinician's practice environment will increase the specificity of the action plans, keep the study focused, and increase the overall usefulness of the results.

There is a strong temptation for clinicians to collect extra data just because they "might be interesting" or because they might be useful for other types of data analyses. Additional data may be interesting, but they may also require additional time to collect. If other types of analyses are to be conducted because they relate to the initial question, then their place in the Model of Rehabilitation Service Delivery should be identified before the study begins, and the rationale should address all of the possible analyses. If additional information is collected for others to study, then the rationale should stay focused on the variables that are included in the initial question. If the clinician cannot identify why specific data are being collected, there is an increased risk of spending time and money obtaining, processing, and analyzing those data.

> *Collecting extra data requires extra time.*

Collecting extra "interesting" data may also require larger sample sizes. The tendency to collect extra data is understandable. After all, if the clinician is already reviewing a chart, why not record another two or three characteristics? The answer is that as the numbers of categories or variables increase, larger samples of patients are needed. and the statistical analyses may become more complicated. Collecting extra data on each patient can increase the time spent on each chart and the time spent finding additional charts to include; both indirectly increase the costs of conducting a study.

> *Collecting "nice to know" but "not essential" data may increase the costs of conducting an outcome study.*

Only the clinician asking the question can decide whether a variable is "essential" or merely "nice to know." By placing the question into the Model for Rehabilitation Service Delivery or the PICO or PIO formats, the clinician is more likely to stay true to the intent of the study. The key to success for those just beginning to learn the steps of outcome measurement is to "keep it simple"; the fewer the variables, the simpler the study!

REASONS FOR CONDUCTING OUTCOME STUDIES

There are four primary reasons for conducting a study: to measure the clinician's own clinical effectiveness, to provide clinician- or setting-specific data to support patient management approaches, to improve the internal management processes of a clinical setting, and to add to the larger body of clinical evidence and knowledge.

Measuring the Clinician's Own Clinical Effectiveness

In keeping with the idea of being a reflective practitioner as described in Chapter 1, each clinician should consider measuring his or her own personal level of effectiveness with patients. When documentation supports the ability to describe trends in patient care management, a clinician can examine objectively how services are delivered and identify areas to strengthen or revise.

> *After new approaches are implemented, objective baselines on practice outcomes allow those outcomes to be compared.*

As new clinical skills are learned and integrated into patient care plans, previous measures of clinical effectiveness allow the clinician to determine if new approaches may be needed. If the initial level of effectiveness has not been quantified before a new approach is implemented, it is difficult to determine if the new approach has made a significant difference in patient outcomes. Consequently, a significant amount of money may be invested to learn a technique but without the ability to determine if the money spent was worthwhile.

Objective measures of a clinician's own patient outcomes facilitate comparison with other clinicians who work with similar groups of patients. This evidence-based comparison, or benchmarking, in a clinical setting is useful for determining who or what approach is more effective—an important step in identifying best practices. Physical therapy has a long history of mentoring by senior clinicians. What is not known is whether seniority is equated with greater clinical effectiveness. That is, do years of experience correlate positively with better clinical outcomes, or is it possible that novice clinicians might approach select patient groups with more efficient interventions? Deference to experience may not be as useful as deference to objective measures of effectiveness, and outcome data comprise that objective measure.

Every clinician should try to answer the question, "How effective am I with patients who have (insert any condition, impairment, or functional limitation)?" Patients like to know if their health-care provider has a good track record and, as consumers, they want to receive cost-effective service. In this era of evidence-based practice, a study that indicates how satisfied patients are with a clinician's service, or how successful a clinician has been in achieving goals within selected diagnoses, goes a long way to providing consumer confidence.

Providing Data to Support Patient Management Decisions

When evidence exists in the literature that a particular intervention or management approach is effective, the ability to deliver that approach and achieve the same outcomes needs to be assessed in each unique clinical setting. Just as patients have unique characteristics that contribute to or detract from the success of a particular intervention, so do clinical practice settings. In addition, when there is no evidence in the literature to guide the clinician, patient data from the clinician's own practice may be the best available evidence to support clinical decision making. Thus, when the study conditions do not match the clinical conditions, or when there are no published data, documentation on the individual patient's response to treatment or from a cohort of patients from the same practice can support clinical decision making.

There are several common reasons why study and clinical conditions do not match. Clinicians are unique to each practice setting. The years of experience, the educational preparation, and the exposure to patient groups may allow some therapists to deliver an intervention more effectively, or just differently, than other therapists. Although it is important that clinical decisions be guided by what is in the literature, the success of any intervention must also be measured across patients to see if the outcomes achieved by individual therapists match those achieved in the literature.

The frequency with which patients receive interventions is another common variable in clinical practice. Inpatients might receive daily services whereas outpatients might receive services one to three times per week. Service delivery in clinical research studies may be provided at higher daily and weekly frequencies or over a longer period than what is typically provided in actual clinical practice. Thus, the effectiveness of an intervention that is supported in the literature may be less effective in clinical practice if that intervention cannot be delivered at the same frequency or with the same intensity as reported in the study's methods.

Finally, the subjects in a published study, for whom an intervention has been shown to be effective, may not closely match the patients receiving the

> *In the absence of published data, data from a specific clinical practice may be useful for supporting clinical decisions.*

> *Different clinicians may yield different results.*

intervention in a clinical setting. The unique inputs that patients bring to the clinical encounter may affect the outcome of any intervention. If patients come from unique demographic regions or from differing cultural backgrounds, or if services are delivered in unusual settings, the patients may not reflect the homogenous patients included in a controlled study.

Providing Data to Support Service Delivery Decisions

Data can be used to support patient management decisions, and they can be used to support administrative service delivery decisions. Outcome studies on patient satisfaction might reveal the need to change administrative processes, such as how patients are scheduled, or the need to provide patients with more education about their care. Outcome data can identify the educational needs of clinical staff, identify administrative procedures that patients are having difficulty with, or determine costs associated with clusters of services. Improvements in any of these areas could ultimately improve service for patients.

Managed care practices have challenged all the ways that health-care services have traditionally been delivered and reimbursed. Outcome studies that address the effects of changes in policy, access to intervention, and the amount of available intervention may be necessary for a particular setting to support its identified best practice or to justify the plan of care for individual patients. Using measurable outcomes allows a clinician to track the changes in practice that are implemented in order to determine if they are better than previous methods. Continuous quality improvement is an ongoing managerial commitment that uses data to direct changes in practice within a particular setting. When changes in practice are applied systematically, the results of those changes can be measured to determine the effectiveness of the changed practice.

Adding to the Larger Body of Knowledge

Clinical sciences are in great need of evidence to support the use of interventions or practice strategies. There are many interventions that are commonly applied in patient care but lack published evidence about their usefulness. The special edition of *Physical Therapy* (October 2001) was devoted to evidence-based guidelines. In all four of the conditions reviewed (low back, knee, neck, and shoulder pain), numerous interventions were examined, for which the conclusion was "evidence for the effectiveness of [intervention] is lacking." These interventions included such common ones as therapeutic ultrasound, massage, and electrical stimulation for acute or chronic low back (p. 1641), knee (p. 1675), neck (p. 1701), and shoulder pain (p. 1719). Outcome studies, even if small in scale, are the building blocks of stronger clinical studies that are needed for sound clinical decision making.

Outcome studies help to clarify "best practice" patterns. In the hustle and bustle of seeing patients, keeping up with documentation, and managing the business of service delivery, it is sometimes difficult to determine what is working well and what is not. Outcome studies that look at departmental procedures or patient outcomes across a group of therapists are helpful for indicating trends in practice. Identifying the most effective trends allows a clinician to analyze how that trend occurs and to systematically alter practice to see if the trend can be strengthened. In contrast, ineffective practices can also be identified and replaced with more effective or efficient activities.

Outcome studies are needed to share the results about the most effective and efficient interventions for different patient groups. When outcome studies are conducted to contribute to the larger body of knowledge, the results are disseminated through publication. This text *does not prepare the reader for a publishable study;* rather, it focuses on a process for measuring the outcomes of an individual clinician for the purposes of improving that clinician's effectiveness in practice.

> ➤ *Published outcome studies help to clarify best practice.*

SUMMARY

Outcome studies require a great deal of energy and commitment, particularly when documentation processes do not allow for easy translation of patient data. In order to make the most effective use of a clinician's efforts, it is critical to know *why* a study is being conducted, not just how to conduct it. A rationale should be specific to the service delivery setting and the practice patterns of the reflective clinician. A clear rationale can help focus the study on the key variables and identify the strategies for change that might improve service delivery. The rationale for conducting the study guides the clinician in the application of data to practice.

References

Philadelphia panel evidence-based clinical practice guidelines on selected rehabilitation interventions for low back pain. (2001). Physical Therapy 91:1641–1674.

Philadelphia panel evidence-based clinical practice guidelines on selected rehabilitation interventions for knee pain. (2001). Physical Therapy 81:1675–1700.

Philadelphia panel evidence-based clinical practice guidelines on selected rehabilitation interventions for neck pain. (2001). Physical Therapy 81:1701–1717.

Philadelphia panel evidence-based clinical practice guidelines on selected rehabilitation interventions for shoulder pain. (2001). Physical Therapy 81:1719–1730.

Coding Data From Clinical Documentation

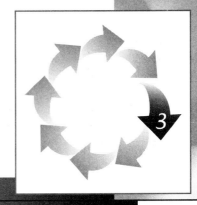

## 9

KEY TERMS

Coding

Disease codes

Impairment codes

Disability codes

Operational definitions

CHAPTER OUTCOMES

➤ Describe the benefits of using coding systems for patient documentation.

➤ Describe the qualities of useful coding systems.

➤ Identify examples of coding systems used in rehabilitation settings.

A coding system is a set of symbols and their definitions used to categorize or organize information about a group of things or people. Code definitions may reflect relative values, such as the coding of levels of strength, or they may be based on mutually exclusive conditions, such as the coding of blood types. Coding systems allow clinicians to read about, document, and compare patient or intervention characteristics using a common language. This chapter will describe the benefits of integrating coding systems into documentation, describe the qualities of useful coding systems, and provide examples of some coding strategies.

THE BENEFITS OF USING A CODING SYSTEM

Medical coding has its origins in the middle 1700s for epidemiological tracking of causes of death (Coiera, 2003). There are many coding systems that describe patient characteristics, and their unique foci influence how patient outcomes are studied. Coding systems are the structural building blocks for data sets because they provide efficient methods of recording detailed clinical information. This section briefly describes the generic benefits and limitations associated with using coding systems in clinical documentation.

Standardization of Terminology

One important benefit of using coding systems is that terminology is standardized for all users. In an evolving profession such as physical therapy, multiple terms have been generated to describe clinical observations. For example, *hyperreflexia, spasticity, hypertonicity*, and *excessive tone* all describe a state of muscle reactivity in people with central nervous system injuries. *Dizziness, vertigo,* and *lightheadedness* are terms used to describe similar perceptions related to vestibular or circulatory impairments.

When multiple terms describe similar phenomena in patient documentation, it becomes difficult to determine whether clinicians are referring to similar or different processes or observations. A coding system links a specific definition to a term or to a set of synonyms, thus differentiating the terms that describe similar but not equivalent observations. Agreement on a single set of terms and definitions allows for standardization of language and of procedures and improves ease of communication. For example, before the Guide to Physical Therapist Practice (1995) was published, clinicians had used the terms *examination* and *evaluation* interchangeably. In the Guide, each term is distinguished by its own definition to reflect a different phase of patient care management. Publication and repeated use of the definitions have clarified communication for a wide range of audiences and consumers.

Reduction of Variability in Documentation

In rehabilitation settings, using a standardized coding system to describe patient conditions reduces variation in patient descriptions and provides common understandings of patient presentations. Within a category (such as strength), there can be multiple levels of terms (such as poor, fair, and normal), each having a minimal performance level defined. By observing or testing a patient, a clinician can identify which performance criteria are met and thus assign a class or rating to the patient's ability level. But if there are multiple definitions or procedures for each term, or there is disagreement among

Using a Classification System

Werneke and Hart's (2003) comparison of centralization classification procedures for patients with low back pain suggests that discriminant validity and relative precision measures are better after multiple visits as compared with after an initial visit for selected patient groups.

staff about which one set of terms or procedures to use, then a single patient record may have the same term reflecting different levels of performance if several clinicians provide documentation.

There are no universally accepted coding systems in rehabilitation. Some systems enjoy greater use because of their historical value, their clarity, their clinical usefulness, or because of their recognition across parties. All coding systems are modifiable and should change as clinical practice advances. It is through testing, application to patient documentation, and further definition of systems' limitations that coding systems improve and become more clinically useful.

Enhanced Completion of Documentation

To use patient documentation to support outcome studies, the documentation needs to be complete. When clinicians agree on a patient coding system, they accept the terms and definitions of measurements and procedures. When everyone agrees on terminology, there is greater likelihood that the measures will be recorded. When there is confusion about terminology, it becomes easier for clinicians to leave items blank (resulting in missing data) or to enter data incorrectly (creating errors in data). In research terms, inter-rater reliability of measurement procedures or definitions improves the chances that the measurements will be taken *and* that they will be documented in the same way by more than one person. If measures are recorded without clear agreement, then the reliability of those measures is compromised. Data that are entered incorrectly, inconsistently, or not at all because of confused interpretations of definitions limit the creation of a useful data set.

Comparison Within Individuals

Coding of patient characteristics allows a clinician to compare patient changes systematically over time. When physical abilities are classified at initial and discharge visits, it is assumed that the conditions and definitions by which the patient is classified are constant. A common characteristic of non-coded documentation is the inconsistency of data on the same behavior or skill. In retrospective chart reviews, it is not uncommon to find that measures recorded at the initial examination may not have been updated on a regular schedule or were not documented as having been measured again at all. When performance criteria are defined for a patient, and the codes for the criteria are integrated into documentation requirements, the results are more frequent repeated measures that describe the patient's recovery. Thus, the adage of comparing apples with apples (or measures with measures) aptly applies to documentation on the same patient characteristics.

Using Repeated Measurements

McClure et al. (2004) used the University of Pennsylvania Shoulder Scale to measure pain, satisfaction, and function before and after 6 weeks of intervention.

Use of a common coding system allows multiple clinicians to document a single patient over time with greater reliability. For example, there are numerous grading scales for strength: some use number ratings, some use letters, some use pluses and minuses, and some do not. If two clinicians are documenting care for the same patient, communication is enhanced if the same codes and definitions are used.

Comparison Across Individuals Within a Setting

One of the greatest advantages of using coding systems is the ability to analyze trends and make comparisons across a group of individuals. Patients with similar characteristics can be studied as groups to measure change within a particular setting. To identify a homogenous patient group, key characteristics of patients need to be coded when the patients are first examined and recoded on subsequent visits if the characteristic changes. These key characteristics can be related to diagnoses, signs and symptoms, scores on tests, or any other measurable or classifiable quality. To create cohort data on similar patient records, several patient characteristics are typically combined to define the eligible group, and the repeated measures of their impairments or functional limitations are harvested to create the data set. This textbook is aimed at this level of outcome study.

Comparison and Collaboration Among Clinical Sites

When a common language is used across sites, data can be combined from multiple sites. Agreement and training in the use of coding systems allow sites to pool data, analyze larger data sets, and compare findings across different types of service delivery models. The International Classification of Function (ICF), formerly the International Classification of Impairments, Disabilities and Handicaps (ICIDH) (1980), is an example of how data can be compared across service delivery models. Many institutions around the world adopted the original ICIDH to describe their patients, and these data sets have been used to describe patterns of care and outcomes across many diagnostic

Classification to Create Equivalent Groups

Tsorlakis et al. (2004) compared two samples of children with cerebral palsy matched by age, sex, and distribution of impairment as categorized by the Gross Motor Function Classification System.

groups. An internationally accepted system of coding allows researchers to explore the differences in patient groups with the same diagnosis and presentation of impairments or functional limitations but who have access to varied amounts of and approaches to health care. The outcomes of similar patients can then be compared to see the importance of different variables.

In addition to revealing differences among data collection sites, common coding systems allow researchers to create larger data sets in less time. When a clinician is interested in a particular type of patient, many months or years may be needed to collect enough patients to create a sample that will yield valid answers. By having several sites pool data using a common coding system, more data for particular patient profiles can be acquired faster. Two successful examples of these types of data sets include the Uniform Data Systems for Medical Rehabilitation, which oversees the collection of FIM data from subacute rehabilitation centers, and FOTO Inc., which oversees collection of data on orthopedic conditions from outpatient physical therapy clinics. Both of these organizations have standardized the data that are collected during patient encounters and have trained clinicians in measurement and data collection processes to ensure reliable measures. Both have created very large data sets that have been analyzed to answer a variety of clinical questions and with which individual institutions can compare their own outcomes.

THE QUALITIES OF USEFUL CODING SYSTEMS

Coding systems are useful only if they describe the subsets of characteristics within a group accurately and reliably. Many different types of coding processes exist in physical therapy practice; however, there are great variations in what is used among clinical settings and within diagnostic groups. As the profession continues to evolve and technology increases its presence in clinical settings, the use of coding systems will increase. Clinicians who are considering adopting coding processes should consider the following.

Operational Definitions

Operational definitions describe both the conceptual idea of a code and the differences among the levels within a code group. They tell others how to use a particular term or measure. This is especially important when multiple terms exist to describe a similar characteristic.

Operational definitions may be detailed enough to include the tools and procedures for measurement of a characteristic (Portney & Watkins, 2000; Rothstein & Echternach, 1993). The purpose of such specificity is to allow others to replicate the measurement procedures accurately and to assign the results to the correct coding label.

Operational Definitions in Research

Fritz et al. (2004, p. 183.) defined patients as having "no improvement" following spinal manipulation if they had 5 or fewer points of improvement on the OSW by the time of the third treatment.

Ideally, operational definitions are found in the literature so that unique, location-specific definitions are not created unnecessarily. Terminology and procedures that have been previously defined often have some level of established reliability. Using established codes provides cleaner comparisons of one study's data with those of others.

When operational definitions do not exist, or when the existing definitions cannot be clearly applied to the conditions observed, new operational definitions may need to be created. If new terms and definitions are created, or if existing codes are being expanded, the reliability of the new operational definitions will need to be tested by having other clinicians apply them.

Mutually Exclusive Categories

The categories of a coding system must be mutually exclusive so that a measurement or characteristic belongs to only one category. If there is an overlap in the category definitions so that the same characteristic qualifies for more than one code, the reliability and usefulness of the system are compromised. For example, most students understand the relative value of achieving a course grade of A rather than a C in a letter grade system. Consider that in some settings the range of scores that qualifies as an A is 89-100. In other settings the range may be 92-100. A student who receives a 90 would qualify for an A in the first setting but not the second. If students from both institutions need to mix, it will be difficult to identify the A students.

Breadth and Depth

A coding system should include the entire range of characteristics it is meant to organize (DeJong, et al., 2004). A system with minimal detail may not be useful, even if it is reliable, if characteristics are missing from the coding options. Likewise, when there is great detail in the coding of one characteristic and absence of codes for other characteristics, the breadth of coding categories limits the collection of useful data. The trick is to find a balance between the number of coded characteristics or measures necessary for outcome documentation and the amount of time that can be devoted to completing forms for other purposes. Adding codes increases documentation time. Even if they provide interesting information, the clinician will need to decide on the most efficient methods for documenting patient status.

Ease of Use

The key to successfully using a coding system in patient documentation is its ease of use. When the coding process is part of the documentation process,

 Operational Definitions in Research

VanSant (1988) created operational definitions to describe body segment movement strategies for the supine-to-stand transition. By refining her operational definitions, she increased inter-tester reliability for the coding process from 90% to 95%.

rather than a separate or parallel process, coding and documentation occur simultaneously. Common reasons for incomplete documentation include lack of time, confusion about what a code means, confusion about who should complete particular forms, and lack of familiarity with selected instruments. When additional coding processes are added to a clinical schedule that already feels tight, the likelihood of completion is diminished unless the coding activities are efficiently integrated into the documentation process.

Computerization of documentation is on the rise in physical therapy and health care in general. More products are available that use a variety of data transfer processes to increase the efficiency and completeness of documentation and coding. Some systems use bubble forms that are read by scanners. Bar code charts can be scanned with a pen reader. Touch screen computers allow information to be entered and coded at the point of care by either the clinician or the consumer. Personal digital assistants are becoming more integrated into full service documentation programs such that coding occurs at the point of service, and data are synchronized with a database accessed through the Internet. As changes in computer electronics continue, the possibilities for patient data collection become more accessible, affordable, and efficient.

There are a number of benefits from using computerized formats for documentation. Translating data from paper-and-pencil documents requires a great deal of time. Someone needs to manually find the charts, go through them page by page to find the relevant characteristics to record, and then manually return the charts. Depending on the number of characteristics that are being studied, the time to find and record the data can be quite extensive, especially if the visit notes are in a narrative format. A computerized record system can be searched by selected variables, and subsets of the data can be constructed with minimal effort.

If a clinician has only paper medical records, standardized forms with dedicated fields for patient information are preferred over SOAP notes or narrative progress notes. Dedicated fields make it easier to retrieve the information because the clinician knows what form to look for and where to find the information on the form. When documentation forms have preprinted codes that can be circled or checked, both documentation efficiency and data retrieval are increased (Fig. 9.1).

Finding the data or patient information in a paper medical record is half the battle, and converting that information into a data set is the other half. Misreading items, miscoding characteristics, or simply coding data from one patient in the sample into someone else's data record because of visual fatigue are all typical human errors that occur when entering large volumes of data. A documentation system that can enter a coded characteristic, measurement, or response to a question into a data set electronically makes that system more time-efficient and reliable.

SOURCES OF CODING CONFUSION

Confusion in coding terminology occurs for several reasons. Terms may differ slightly but have the same operational definitions, such as the words *examination* and *evaluation*. As mentioned earlier, these terms had been interchangeable until the Guide to Physical Therapist Practice (1997) provided a common taxonomy with operational definitions. Now they have come to mean distinctly different processes.

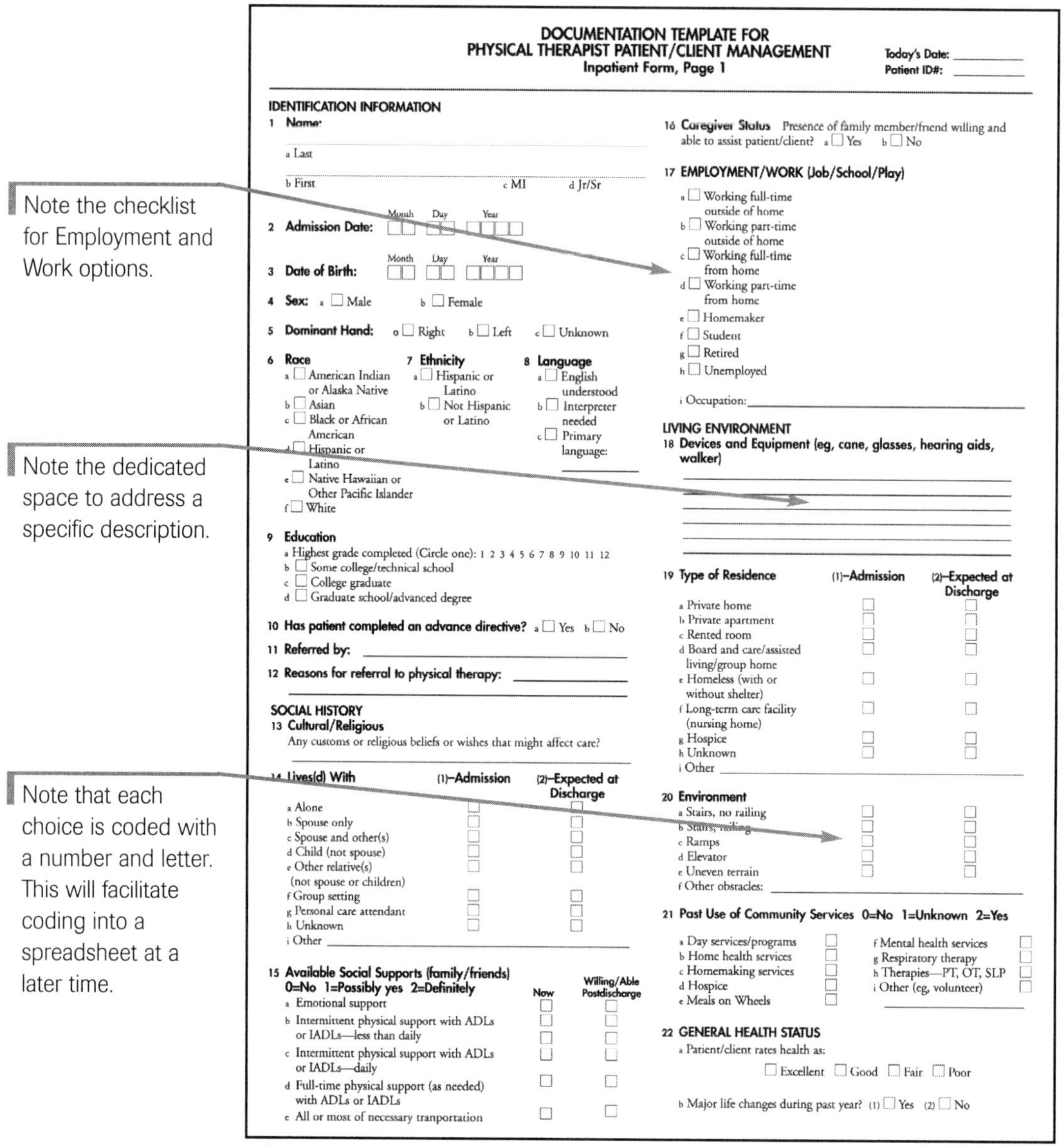
Note the checklist for Employment and Work options.
Note the dedicated space to address a specific description.
Note that each choice is coded with a number and letter. This will facilitate coding into a spreadsheet at a later time.

DOCUMENTATION TEMPLATE FOR
PHYSICAL THERAPIST PATIENT/CLIENT MANAGEMENT
Inpatient Form, Page 1

Today's Date: ________
Patient ID#: ________

IDENTIFICATION INFORMATION
1 Name:
a Last
b First c MI d Jr/Sr
2 Admission Date: Month Day Year
3 Date of Birth: Month Day Year
4 Sex: a ☐ Male b ☐ Female
5 Dominant Hand: a ☐ Right b ☐ Left c ☐ Unknown
6 Race
a ☐ American Indian or Alaska Native
b ☐ Asian
c ☐ Black or African American
d ☐ Hispanic or Latino
e ☐ Native Hawaiian or Other Pacific Islander
f ☐ White
7 Ethnicity
a ☐ Hispanic or Latino
b ☐ Not Hispanic or Latino
8 Language
a ☐ English understood
b ☐ Interpreter needed
c ☐ Primary language: ________
9 Education
a Highest grade completed (Circle one): 1 2 3 4 5 6 7 8 9 10 11 12
b ☐ Some college/technical school
c ☐ College graduate
d ☐ Graduate school/advanced degree
10 Has patient completed an advance directive? a ☐ Yes b ☐ No
11 Referred by: ________
12 Reasons for referral to physical therapy: ________

SOCIAL HISTORY
13 Cultural/Religious
Any customs or religious beliefs or wishes that might affect care?
14 Lives(d) With (1)–Admission (2)–Expected at Discharge
a Alone
b Spouse only
c Spouse and other(s)
d Child (not spouse)
e Other relative(s) (not spouse or children)
f Group setting
g Personal care attendant
h Unknown
i Other ________
15 Available Social Supports (family/friends) 0=No 1=Possibly yes 2=Definitely — Now / Willing/Able Postdischarge
a Emotional support
b Intermittent physical support with ADLs or IADLs—less than daily
c Intermittent physical support with ADLs or IADLs—daily
d Full-time physical support (as needed) with ADLs or IADLs
e All or most of necessary tranportation

16 Caregiver Status Presence of family member/friend willing and able to assist patient/client? a ☐ Yes b ☐ No
17 EMPLOYMENT/WORK (Job/School/Play)
a ☐ Working full-time outside of home
b ☐ Working part-time outside of home
c ☐ Working full-time from home
d ☐ Working part-time from home
e ☐ Homemaker
f ☐ Student
g ☐ Retired
h ☐ Unemployed
i Occupation: ________

LIVING ENVIRONMENT
18 Devices and Equipment (eg, cane, glasses, hearing aids, walker)
19 Type of Residence (1)–Admission (2)–Expected at Discharge
a Private home
b Private apartment
c Rented room
d Board and care/assisted living/group home
e Homeless (with or without shelter)
f Long-term care facility (nursing home)
g Hospice
h Unknown
i Other ________
20 Environment
a Stairs, no railing
b Stairs, railing
c Ramps
d Elevator
e Uneven terrain
f Other obstacles: ________
21 Past Use of Community Services 0=No 1=Unknown 2=Yes
a Day services/programs
b Home health services
c Homemaking services
d Hospice
e Meals on Wheels
f Mental health services
g Respiratory therapy
h Therapies—PT, OT, SLP
i Other (eg, volunteer)
22 GENERAL HEALTH STATUS
a Patient/client rates health as: ☐ Excellent ☐ Good ☐ Fair ☐ Poor
b Major life changes during past year? (1) ☐ Yes (2) ☐ No

Figure 9.1 Example of a form with dedicated fields and checklist items. (From the APTA Guide to Physical Therapist Practice [1997].)

Terms may be the same but are defined differently across settings or diagnoses. The term *disability* refers to the presence of *impairments* in the 1990 Americans with Disabilities Act P.L. 101-336, *functional limitations* in the 1980 version of the International Classification of Impairments, Disabilities and Handicaps, and *social limitations* in the National Agenda for Prevention of Disabilities (Iezzoni, 2002). Thus, depending on the model of disablement that is used, the same term can refer to very different constructs (Iezzoni, 2002; Jette, 1995; US Dept. of Health and Human Services, 1993).

Terms may have definitions that do not fit the reality of the situation or do not accurately describe an observation or behavior the clinician wants to measure. For example, the term *independent toileting* may not realistically imply total independence from adult supervision when talking about preschoolers. When terms are confusing or lack appropriate descriptions to suit the situation, it may be necessary to create new terms or definitions. In any case, it is the clinician's responsibility to identify terminology that has been adequately tested for its usefulness or to test new terms that are created before using them in documentation.

EXAMPLES OF CODING SYSTEMS

There are numerous coding systems used in rehabilitation settings; this section describes some of them. These systems represent attempts to standardize a variety of patient care characteristics and processes. The choice of system will depend on the clinical setting requirements, the types and purposes of the outcomes to be studied, the practicality of collecting data, and the amount of support available for managing the data. In some cases, a clinic may already be using a system to organize data, but the data may not be easily retrievable. In other settings, the data may be quite available with little effort. In settings that do not use electronic records, the data may be available only by manually reviewing patient charts and converting narrative reports into coded data. When starting an outcome study, the clinician will need to determine what coded information is already accessible and useful for answering the question of choice.

The following examples are provided as an overview of what can be used. This is not an exhaustive list. As practice evolves, it is important to check for updates or newly created coding systems.

Disease Coding

Diseases and injuries can be classified with multiple methods: by the cause (gunshot wounds), by the pathology (coronary artery disease), or by the presentation of symptoms (fevers with rashes). Often, the coding aids administrative processes, such as ICD-10 codes, and is used by institutions and government agencies for patient tracking, billing processes, utilization management, and quality improvement initiatives.

Administrative codes may be useful for creating sample groups to study, but there are several limitations to using them for outcome studies. The data are often plagued by inconsistent applications of codes, lack of coding for coexisting conditions that the patient is not being treated for at the time, lack of sensitivity to the patient's health status or level of severity of a diagnosis, and lack of reference to functional status (Iezzoni, 2002). Thus, if administrative codes are used to create a sample of patients who have the same diagnosis, it will not be known if the members of that sample have the same levels of severity or functional limitations. Nevertheless, the coding systems are in place and are typically integrated into documentation processes. If they are used for creating sample sets, the clinician may want to consider additional characteristics or codes to ensure homogeneity of the study sample.

ICD-10

The International Classification of Diseases, 10th Revision (ICD-10), is a set of codes for reporting morbidity and mortality statistics around the world. The ICD-10 belongs to a body of international classification schema organized by the World Health Organization, but the codification of diseases and causes of death dates back to the mid-1700s (who.int/classifications/icd/en/).

ICD-9-CM

The International Classification of Diseases, Ninth Revision, Clinical Modification (ICD-9-CM) provides a coding system of diseases and interventions for hospital inpatients, outpatients, and physician office visits. The coding supports data for medical records and case reviews, ambulatory and other medical care programs, and for basic health statistics. It is based on the WHO international ICD-9 (who.int/whosis/icd10/othercla.htm). The National Center for Health Statistics and the Centers for Medicare and Medicaid Services are the agencies responsible for annual updates and modifications to the codes in the United States (cdc.gov/nchs/about/otheract/icd9/abticd9.htm).

DSM-IV-TR

The Diagnostic and Statistical Manual of Mental Disorders, Fourth Edition, Text Revision (DSM-IV-TR) (2000) is a coding system for mental health disorders published by the American Psychiatric Association. It includes criteria and descriptions to guide the coding process (behavenet.com/capsules/disorders/dsm4tr.htm).

Impairment Coding

In general, impairments are the patient characteristics in physical therapy practice that are measured most often. Many impairments, such as limited range of motion or strength, are measured with an instrument or scale. Because most impairments are defined by a measurable quality, there is no need to create a separate code. In fact, it is preferable to enter the raw measurements rather than transcribe them into larger, less defined, categories. For example, it would be preferable to record the actual degrees of range of motion rather than translate them into a less accurate category of mild or moderate limitation. Data entered in their raw form lend themselves to multiple types of analyses that cannot be performed on transcribed data. Transcribing data into larger, thematic categories can always be done after the raw data are recorded.

Impairment documentation is quite prevalent in physical therapy. The following are common examples of impairment along with measures that lend themselves easily to standardized reporting processes.

- Strength: recorded as dynamometer readings or as manual muscle test grades
- Range of motion: recorded as degrees of movement
- Pain: recorded in millimeters on a visual analog scale
- Wound size: recorded as the diameter or with a wound classification scale (Armstrong, Lavery, & Harkless, 1998)

In each of these examples, operational definitions are available to describe measures or levels within the category. When possible, use a measurement that results in a number. For some coding schemas, like manual muscle testing, there may be several documented versions of strength categories. In this case, the clinician will need to determine which one to use consistently. It is preferable to use measures or codes that have established reliability so as to avoid creation of new, untested codes. But whether the codes have been tested for reliability or not, the clinician should conduct some training and testing sessions to achieve an acceptable level of reliability for the chosen codes.

Disability Coding

There are many models of disablement that provide operational definitions of the terminology related to the problems patients face as a consequence of disease or injury. (See Chapter 5 for a review of various models.) These models of disablement provide organizing terminology for a growing body of measurement tools that look at aspects of patient status other than the impairments. The limitation of using a model to classify patient management is that there may not be established gradations, categories, or codes defined within each of the larger components of the model, and without published codes data sets are individualized to each clinical setting. One notable exception to this limitation is the International Classification of Function (ICF), which provides both a model of disablement and a coding system to describe patient status.

> *Impairment measures, such as range of motion limitations, are most useful if entered as the raw measurement of degrees rather than translated into less specific categories of limitation (e.g., mildly or moderately limited).*

ICF (Formerly ICIDH)

The International Classification of Impairments, Disabilities and Handicaps (ICIDH) was published by the World Health Organization in 1980. This system established a letter and numerical code system for a wide variety of impairments or body level restrictions, disabilities or task level restrictions, and handicaps or social role restrictions that occur as a consequence of disease. Countries around the world have been using the coding system to describe patients, allowing the ability to track disablement trends across nations. The ICIDH underwent a 9-year international revision process that resulted in the ICF (2001), which updates language, provides greater specificity, broadens the types of categories used to describe the consequences of disease, and places a new emphasis on abilities as well as limitations.

The ICF is organized around two major parts. Part 1 contains the coding domains of Body Functions, Body Structures, and Activities and Participation in real life. Part 2 contains the domains of environmental and personal factors; however, there are no codes associated with the personal factors. Each domain is structured as a hierarchy, with coding letters and numbers assigned to set locations. The first letter in a code series identifies the domain related to the problem: b… represents codes from Body Functions, s… represents codes from Body Structures, d… represents codes from Activities and Participation, which can be listed separately as a… and p…, respectively. Codes representing the domain of Environment begin with e….

Following the letter code for the domain is a second-level, 1-digit numerical code for the chapter that lists additional codes for the problem. A code of s7… would refer to a body structure problem related to movement. A code of d4… represents a problem with activities; more specifically, a problem with mobility.

Following the domain letter and the chapter code comes a two-digit code representing greater detail about the nature of the problem. A code of d420 represents a problem with activities and participation, from the ICF Chapter 4 on Mobility, specifically problems with transferring oneself.

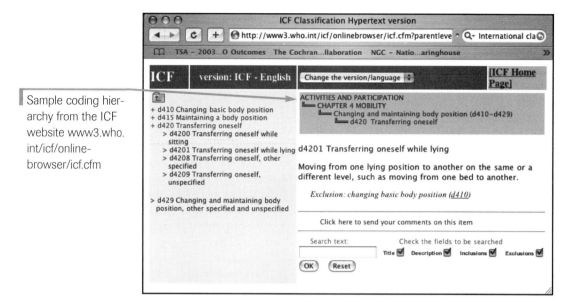

Sample coding hierarchy from the ICF website www3.who.int/icf/online-browser/icf.cfm

Figure 9.2 Sample coding hierarchy from the ICF website. (From World Health Organization [2005]:http://www3.who.int/icf/onlinebrowser/icf.com.)

A fifth numerical code provides even greater detail about the activity that is limited. Following the previous example, a code d4201 refers to a problem with transferring oneself from one lying position to another lying position. In contrast, a code d4200 refers to a problem with transferring oneself from one sitting position to another (Fig. 9.2).

Following the five-digit code is a decimal place holder, and two to three additional modifying codes, depending on the domain. Body structure codes have three modifiers that may follow the decimal point, representing the extent of the change (none to complete impairment), the nature of the change, and the location of the impairment (right or left, proximal or distal). Activities and participation have two to four levels of qualifiers, the first representing performance quality and the second representing the capacity to perform. The optional third and fourth qualifiers relate to performance with and without assistance.

The five-digit coding process (up to the decimal point, or the four-level code as it is called in the ICF) provides 1424 distinct codes to describe the problems that a patient might have as a consequence of disease. The ICF manual suggests that two-level codes might be appropriate for survey and health outcome studies and that the four-level codes are more appropriate for specialist services, including rehabilitation.

The interactive online versions of the ICF can be accessed at the website for the World Health Organization at www3.who.int/icf/icftemplate.cfm. Hard copies of the books may also be ordered from the same address. Clinicians should be aware of this tool because it represents an international, validated coding system that can be used to describe the array of problems with which any patient might present. A child version of the ICF is under development and can also be viewed at the website. The APTA is currently participating in a multidisciplinary process to develop a clinician user manual for the ICF to enhance its use across professions.

Minimum Data Set

The Minimum Data Set (MDS) is administered by Medicare and contains quarterly data collected through the Resident Assessment Instrument (cms.hhs.gov/quality/mds20/) about patients from nursing homes. This cross-sectional survey of nursing home residents contains data on patient tracking and demographics, admission dates, items about the patient's routine level of functioning prior to admission, and admission status in many areas including communication, well-being, activities of daily living (ADL) functions, and mobility skills. The data are used primarily for adjusting the reimbursement rates for nursing home care. Because the MDS includes both diagnostic codes and ratings of health status (e.g., cognition, physical functioning, and daily activities), it may be more useful for identifying trends across groups. The primary limitation of this data set is that it does not follow individuals over time but rather samples the resident population four times per year.

OASIS

The Outcome and Assessment Information Set is also administered by Medicare and is collected on all patients who receive home health care. It is also an administrative coding process used to determine reimbursement rates for home care and for quality improvement initiatives (cms.hhs.gov/oasis/hhoview.asp). It codes information on a variety of impairments, disability, and social limitations.

Unified Parkinson Disease Rating Scale

The Unified Parkinson Disease Rating Scale (UPDRS) is an example of a disease-specific rating tool used to describe levels of disability in patients with Parkinson's disease. It has three major components (mentation, ADLs, and motor) that combine questions about impairments and functional limitations to determine levels of disability. It provides the user with a numerical score ranging from 199 for maximal disability to 0 representing no disability (National Parkinson Foundation, 2006).

PEDI

The Pediatric Evaluation of Disability Inventory is an example of an age-related tool that is not diagnosis-specific. It is a parent-report questionnaire about the functional abilities of children, ages 6 months to 7 years (Feldman, Haley, & Coryell, 1990). It measures aspects of functional status: actual functional abilities, caregiver assistance, and modifications of tasks by changes in the environment or use of adaptive equipment. It looks at three major domains: self-care skills, mobility, and social functions.

Intervention Coding

Systems for classifying patient characteristics and the outcomes of intervention are far more available than systems to classify interventions. The ability to describe effective practice rests on the ability to track the interventions that are delivered. Randomized controlled clinical trials (RCTs) are considered the strongest method for establishing the effectiveness of a treatment, but RCTs are conducted under highly controlled conditions. In clinical practice, multiple interventions are combined during the management of a patient so the effect of each treatment is not as clear. When studying the clinical outcomes of interventions, it would be useful to identify the clusters of interventions delivered. Two methods of intervention coding are described below.

CPT Codes

Common Procedural Terms (CPT) are numerical codes assigned to medical procedures. They are administrative codes used primarily for billing third party payers and are often used by departments to describe the frequency of interventions that clinicians provide. CPT codes were originally designed for physician use, so the level of detail and content validity for physical therapy procedures does not represent the scope of what physical therapists provide. Although more codes have been added over the years, they still lack the breadth and depth of detail that is necessary to describe the true array of physical therapy interventions. Even though a lack of content validity is a primary limitation, CPT codes are currently part of routine documentation for many clinical settings. As such, they are available for use in outcome studies, but interpretations of outcomes should be guarded.

The National Classification of Physiotherapy Practice 2000

The Finnish Hospital League published an English version of the Terminology of Physiotherapy in 1993; it is a classification of the types of physiotherapy intervention procedures that are typically performed with patients. The classification was revised in 2000 and pilot-tested in 2002 (2003). This system groups activities into six major categories of activities with a three-digit coding system. The first digit reflects the six categories of intervention:

F1. Physiotherapeutic Examination and Assessment

F2. Counseling and Therapeutic Activities in Physiotherapy

F3. Physiotherapy Services Supporting Clients in their Living and Working Environment

F4. Indirect Physiotherapy for Clients

F5. Expertise and Education Activities

F9. Administration and Internal Development Work

The second and third digits within each major category further define the types of activities within it (Fig. 9.3). To date, this is the only known system of coding developed that reflects the breadth of physical therapy clinical practice. Holma and Noronen (2003) presented pilot outcome data from 20 physiotherapists in 4 settings, demonstrating that the classification system is useful for standardizing language and for describing time allocation among settings and individual clinicians.

The National Classification of Physiotherapy Practice 2000
Free translation from Finnish by Leena Noronen 24.5.2003

THE MAIN CATEGORIES, SUBCATEGORIES AND THE SINGLE MEANS AND METHODS OF THE CLASSIFICATION

F1   PHYSIOTHERAPEUTIC EXAMINATION AND ASSESSMENT

F110 Physiotherapeutic assessment for orientation

F120 Physiotherapeutic assessment
F121   Assessment of functioning and workability
F122   Assessment of physical capacity
F123   Assessment of control over and coordination of positions and movements
F124   Assessment of pain
F130 Writing the physiotherapy plan

F190 Other physiotherapeutic examination and assessment

F2   COUNSELLING AND THERAPEUTIC ACTIVITIES IN PHYSIOTHERAPY

F210 Physiotherapeutic guidance and counselling
F211   Counselling in health promotion
F212   Guidance and counselling in promoting functioning
F213   Guidance and counselling in promoting workability
F214   Writing the individual physiotherapy programme

F220 Therapeutic exercises
F221   Exercising functional capacity and mobility
F222   Exercising physical capacity
F223   Exercising control over and coordination of positions and movements

F230 Manual therapy
F231   Soft tissue treatment
F232   Mobilisation and stabilisation of joint
F233   Joint manipulation

F240 Electrical and thermal procedures
F241   Thermal procedures
F242   Electrical procedures

F290 Other counselling and therapeutic activities in physiotherapy

F3   PHYSIOTHERAPY SERVICES SUPPORTING CLIENTS IN THEIR LIVING AND WORKING ENVIRONMENT

F310 Services supporting movement and functional capacity with assistive devices
F311   Assessment, planning and follow-up of the need for assistive devices
F312   Choosing and providing assistive devices
F313   Loaning, guiding and training to use assistive devices
F314   Actions needed for reparation and maintenance of assistive devices

F320 Services supporting management in domestic life and living environment
F321   Assessment of management in the living environment
F322   Alterations in living environment
F323   Services supporting the control over environment

F330 Physiotherapy services supporting management at work
F331   Assessment of work performance
F332   Preventive and remedial activities

F390 Other services supporting management in domestic life and living environment

F4   INDIRECT PHYSIOTHERAPY FOR CLIENTS

F410 Knowledge acquisition

F420 Documentation
F421   Documentation in patient/ client records
F422   Writing the feed-back or reports on physiotherapy

F430 Multiprofessional collaboration
F431   Cooperation in the treatment of the client
F432   Participation in planning of rehabilitation
F433   Organising continuity of physiotherapy for a client
F434   Physiotherapy as a part of multiprofessional counselling or therapy

F440 Physiotherapist´s consultation

F490 Other indirect physiotherapy for clients

F5   EXPERTISE AND EDUCATION ACTIVITIES

F510 Acting as an expert

F520 Educational activities
F521   Acting as an educator
F522   Work guidance and acquaintance activities
F523   Guidance for other personnel

F530 Student guidance
F531   Guidance for physiotherapy students
F532   Guidance for other students

F540 Producing written material
F541   Producing material for physiotherapeutic use
F542   Writing publications, articles and reports

F590 Other expertise and education activities

F9   ADMINISTRATION AND INTERNAL DEVELOPMENT WORK

F910 Administrative activities
F920 Further education
F930 Research and development work
F940 Quality management
F950 Marketing and information
F990 Other administration and internal development work

Figure 9.3 The National Classification of Physiotherapy Practice 2000. (Reprinted with permission from T. Holma on behalf of The Association of Finnish Local and Regional Authorities.)

CODING DATA FROM NARRATIVE NOTES

Outcome data can be harvested from a wide variety of patient documentation formats. These formats may vary from electronic records, to highly structured sets of patient information forms and examination flow sheets, to loosely structured collections of narrative notes on patients. Some record systems may use a combination of these formats.

This textbook is focused on retrospective data collection; that is, collection of data from previously existing records. The coding systems described in the previous section may already be in use as part of the documentation standards of a particular clinic. If so, then the clinician will have an easier time creating a data set because a coding system has already standardized the way selected patient characteristics are documented.

If there are no coding systems used as part of standard practice, the clinician may find it useful to translate patient documentation into coded data using one of the existing coding paradigms or by creating a new one. For example, the problem list from an initial examination may be easily transcribed into coded data using the ICF codes. The clinician will need to keep meticulous records of the decision-making process for selecting codes so that patient records transcribed at later date have the codes reliably applied.

If the coding systems that are in place are not adequate, or if there are no standardized coding systems in place, it may be necessary to create a coding system to meet the needs of a particular question. In this case, the clinician will need to establish the coding definitions for the variables of interest and then pilot-test them on several charts to see if patient notes can be transcribed without confusion by using the operational definitions.

SUMMARY

Coding is the process of converting observations to alphanumeric representations for data entry. Coding patient characteristics allows clinicians to track changes within patients and across patient groups. Documentation systems incorporate varying amounts of coding, with narrative documents having the least amount of coded information, and computerized documents having the greatest amount. Useful coding systems have clear operational definitions, mutually exclusive categories, and enough depth and breadth to represent the observations accurately, and should be easy to use. Examples of coding systems for pathology, impairment, disability, and intervention demonstrate methods for standardizing the recording of patient information. Coding that is prospectively integrated into clinical documentation provides the most efficient access to patient data for retrospective studies; however, narrative notes can be transcribed into coded data for retrospective studies using existing coding paradigms.

References

American Physical Therapy Association (1995). A guide to physical therapist practice, vol. 1: A description of patient management. Physical Therapy 75(8):707–756.

American Physical Therapy Association (1997). Guide to Physical Therapist Practice. American Physical Therapy Association, Alexandria, VA.

American Physical Therapy Association (2001). Guide to physical therapist practice, 2nd ed.

American Physical Therapy Association, Alexandria, VA.

American Psychiatric Association (2000). Diagnostic and Statistical Manual of Mental Disorders, Fourth Edition, Text Revision (DSM-IV-TR). Arlington, VA.

Armstrong DG, Lavery LA, & Harkless LB (1998). Validation of a diabetic wound classification system. Diabetes Care 21(5):855–859.

Coiera E (2003). Healthcare Terminologies and Classification Systems in Guide to Health Informatics, 2nd ed. Oxford University Press.

DeJong G, et al. (2004). Toward a taxonomy of rehabilitation interventions: Using an inductive approach to examine the "Black Box" of rehabilitation. Archives of Physical Medicine and Rehabilitation 85:678–686.

Feldman AB, Haley SM, & Coryell J (1990). Concurrent and construct validity of the Pediatric Evaluation of Disability Inventory. Physical Therapy 70(10):602–610.

Focus on Therapeutic Outcomes, Inc. (FOTO) P.O. Box 11444, Knoxville, Tennessee 37939–1444.

Fritz JM, et al. (2004). Factors related to the inability of individuals with low back pain to improve with a spinal manipulation. Physical Therapy 84(2):173–190.

Holma T & Noronen L (2003). The National Classification of Physiotherapy Practice: Continuous tool development: A never-ending story? (abstract). World Confederation of Physical Therapy.

Iezzoni LI (2002). Using administrative data to study persons with disabilities. The Milbank Quarterly 80(2):347–379.

Jette AM (1995). Outcomes research: Shifting the dominant research paradigm in physical therapy. Physical Therapy 75:965–970.

McClure PW, et al. (2004). Shoulder function and 3-dimensional kinematics in people with shoulder impingement syndrome before and after a 6-week exercise program. Physical Therapy 84(9):832–848.

Portney LG & Watkins MP (2000). The research question. In Foundations of Clinical Research: Applications to Practice. Prentice Hall Health, Upper Saddle River, NJ.

Rothstein JM & Echternach JL (1993). The basics: terms and concepts. In Primer on Measurement: An Introductory Guide to Measurement Issues. APTA, Alexandria, VA.

Tsorlakis N, Evaggelinou C, Grouios G, & Tsorbatzoudis C (2004). Effect of intensive neurodevelopmental treatment in gross motor function of children with cerebral palsy. Developmental Medicine and Child Neurology 46(11):740–745.

The Finnish Hospital League (1993). Terminology of physiotherapy. Helsinki, Finland.

Uniform Data System for Medical Rehabilitation, 270 Northpointe Parkway, Suite 300, Amherst, NY 14228.

US Dept. of Health and Human Services (1993). Research plan for the National Center for Medical Rehabilitation Research. NIH Pub. No. 93–3509.

VanSant AF (1988). Rising from a supine position to erect stance: Description of adult movement and a developmental hypothesis. Physical Therapy 68(2):185–192.

Werneke M & Hart DL (2003). Discriminant validity and relative precision of classifying patients with nonspecific neck and back pain by anatomic pain patterns. Spine 28:161–166.

World Health Organization (2001). International classification of functioning, disability and health: ICF. Geneva, Switzerland.

Websites

BehaveNet Clinical Capsule: DSM-IV-TR (2005). Diagnostic and statistical manual of mental disorders, 4th ed. (behavenet.com/capsules/disorders/dsm4tr.htm)

Centers for Medicare and Medicaid Services (2005). MDS 2.0 Information Site (cms.hhs.gov/medicaid/mds20/)

—(2005). Chapter 3 - Item-by-Item Guide to the MDS in the RAI User's Manual by Chapter. (cms.hhs.gov/quality/mds20)

—(2005). OASIS Overview. (cms.hhs.gov/oasis/hhoview.asp)

The National Center for Health Statistics (2005). Classification of diseases, functioning and disability: ICD9-CM. (cdc.gov/nchs/about/otheract/icd9/abticd9.htm)

World Health Organization (2005): Classification: History of the ICD (who.int/classifications/icd/en/)

National Parkinson Foundation (2006) (parkinson.org/site/pp.asp?c=9dJFJLPwB&b=123510)

Constructing the Data Set

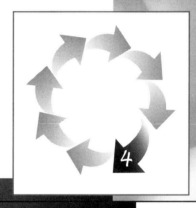

## 10

KEY TERMS

Data set

Spreadsheet

Flat files

Rows

Columns

Cells

Relational database

Transformed data

Data recording form

Coding handbook

CHAPTER OUTCOMES

➤ Identify the basic components and terminology of data sets.

➤ Describe the differences between a flat file and a relational database.

➤ Apply coding knowledge and tips for entering data into a spreadsheet.

This chapter introduces data set terminology, two formats in which data can be stored, and the basic components of a spreadsheet. Examples of typical clinical data illustrate how to categorize data, how to assign codes, and how to enter data into a simple spreadsheet. The basic components of a data set are introduced for readers who have no familiarity with them. Readers who are familiar with data sets from statistics courses, spreadsheet packages, or database software may want to skip to the section The Coding Handbook (p.147).

THE BASIC COMPONENTS OF A DATA SET

A **data set** is a collection of data organized according to selected characteristics. It is a general term that refers to a collection of numerical and/or text data. There are two ways to store data sets; as flat files or relational files. Flat files are simpler to organize and are adequate for smaller data sets. Relational files require a little more planning and software knowledge but offer more flexibility in analyzing larger or more complicated data sets.

Spreadsheets

Spreadsheets are flat files. They are two-dimensional data organization tools consisting of rows and columns that are designed to handle numerical data but can also accommodate text labels. Spreadsheets are generally not efficient for manipulating text-based data, but they are excellent for conducting mathematical functions on numerical data. The study variables are organized across the top of each column, and the rows represent the different cases or patients. The size of the data set grows in width as the variables increase or in length as the cases increase.

Spreadsheets can be created with paper and pencil, and calculations can be done manually. Electronic spreadsheets have integrated data management functions in the software. Text data are typically converted to numerical codes to facilitate analyses. Examples of commercially available spreadsheet software packages include Microsoft Excel, Lotus 1-2-3, and AppleWorks.

One advantage of a flat file is the simplicity of creating the data set. As a study is developed and the relevant characteristics are determined, new variables can be added as they are identified. For example, suppose a clinician developed a data set that included patient referral sources, demographics, initial evaluation measurements, discharge measurements, and patient satisfaction scores. If the clinician later decides that another variable should be added to the spreadsheet, such as pre- and post-treatment quality-of-life scores, new columns can easily be added to the data set.

A second advantage of a flat file is that it is possible to view all the sample data simultaneously. This is especially helpful for spotting trends and errors in the data after all the data points are entered.

The primary disadvantage of a flat file is that large data sets become difficult to manage. Entering data on many variables creates excessively wide data sets. When the data sets are wide, spreadsheet pages are added to the right, which makes it more difficult to see all the pertinent data at one time. It is also easier to enter data into the wrong place when there are large numbers of variable columns, thus introducing errors into the data set. If a single, large spreadsheet with all patients and all variable columns is opened each time clerical information needs to be entered, the possibility of entering

	Variable 1	Variable 2	Variable 3
Subject 1			
Subject 2			
Subject 3			
Subject 4			
Subject 5			
Subject 6			

Figure 10.1 Skeleton of a simple spreadsheet.

information under the wrong variable or wrong patient record is increased. Figure 10.1 illustrates the skeleton of a basic spreadsheet.

Relational Databases

Relational databases are multidimensional organizational tools that can accommodate both numerical and text data. New data are entered through a standardized format of fields into which responses are typed or selected from menus. Prompts at designated character fields cue the typist so that only predetermined formats of data are accepted. Databases accept text data more easily than spreadsheets and allow more flexible management of larger data sets. Due to the standardized format of fields, multiple users can enter data with greater reliability. This is especially useful in clinical settings where clerical staff, clinicians, and patients all may contribute to a centralized data set. Electronic merging of data from multiple sources minimizes the labor costs and opportunities for error that can occur when data are transcribed manually from paper records. Examples of commercially available database software include dBase V, Visual FoxPro, and Microsoft Access.

Relational files can be considered a series of flat files linked by one or more common identifying characteristics. In most cases, the identifier is a patient number that is assigned for all documentation processes (e.g., scheduling, billing, data collection). The identifying number allows different types of data to be kept in separate spreadsheets, which can simplify data entry and management. The identifier also allows for items from separate spreadsheets to be recombined into a new spreadsheet for analysis. This means that a spreadsheet will contain only the data for the patients and the variables related to a specific question, rather than all data on all patients. Figure 10.2 illustrates how several spreadsheets might be organized and linked. Each box represents a different spreadsheet with its column headings.

In this example, the **ID number** is the common identifying characteristic, appearing in each spreadsheet. This ID number is assigned when the patient registers on the first visit, and it is entered on all forms that are completed by the patient or the clinician who works with the patient. Although it is possible to enter all this information into a single flat file, this example illustrates three advantages of the relational database.

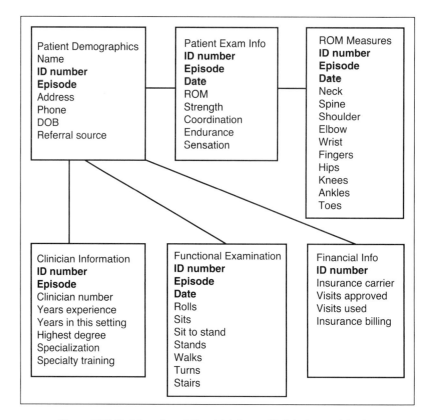

Figure 10.2 Skeleton of a relational database with linked spreadsheets.

The first advantage is that the size of each component spreadsheet is smaller, because information is organized by categories. Patient demographic information, often collected by clerical staff, would be collected in one spreadsheet. Data entered by a clinician is linked to one of several spreadsheets, depending on the content and amount of detail needed. Financial information would be organized in another spreadsheet. When a person needs to enter data, pulling up the part of a file limited to the pertinent information and having labeled fields as prompts reduce the possibility of data being entered into the wrong place.

Relational databases also make it easier to track information about a patient across an episode of care for one problem and across episodes of care for the same or another problem. Layers of spreadsheets can be linked, and the complexity of data that can be managed is far greater than in a flat file. For example, a patient may require rehabilitation services first for one injury and later for a different injury. The additional identifying characteristic of **Episode** allows a clinician to identify a single start date that links all other data related to the first episode by that same date, and a second start date links the data for the second injury. Now a clinician can view the data for a specific type of injury across many patients or view one patient's history over different episodes of care.

Relational data sets allow the user to explode details recorded on a particular characteristic. In Figure 10.2, the data in the Patient Exam Info box would need to be limited to a single code that could be entered for each quality listed. For example, range of motion (ROM) is listed as a quality. If only one code can be listed in a column under that name, the code would need to answer a very basic or global question. Any of the following three coding options could be used, but there is room for only one code.

Code option 1:   Are there ROM limitations?
                  1 = Yes
                  2 = No

Code option 2:   Where are there ROM limitations?
                  1 = None   2 = LU   3 = RUE
                  4 = LLE   5 = RLE   6 = LU&LE
                  7 = RU&LE   8 = Neck/Spine 9 = All limbs

Code option 3:   To what degree are there ROM limitations?
                  1 = None
                  2 = Mild
                  3 = Moderate
                  4 = Severe

The levels of detail provided limit all three coding options. In a relational database, a separate file of data can be linked with the exact ROM measurements recorded for a specified episode of care. In Figure 10.2 the ROM category in Patient Exam Info might be coded using Option 1, but there is also a related data set, entitled "ROM Measures," that specifically stores ROM measurements organized by each episode of care and date of measurement. Given the ability to combine information and explode the detail when it is appropriate, a patient's ROM measurements recorded a year earlier or recorded at the initial examination can be compared with current ROM measures to assess the changes.

In summary, the advantages of a relational database are the ability to collect larger amounts of data, organized by linking smaller files or spreadsheets that are category-specific, with greater reliability among multiple users. The amount of detail that can be organized on a single patient becomes limitless, as all the spreadsheets are linked. Whereas flat files and relational databases allow the investigator to combine specific categories of data to analyze, relational databases are more efficient at manipulating large sets of data.

The primary limitations of a relational database result from the clinician's comfort with database software and the need to plan the types of data to be collected before designing the database. For the clinician who is just beginning to organize data for self-reflection, a flat file format will be adequate. For a clinical department looking to organize data on patients so that future outcome studies can be conducted, a relational database is better suited to handle the number of cases and diverse types of information that can be collected.

THE CODING HANDBOOK

Regardless of whether a paper or an electronic data set will be constructed, there are steps that can be taken prior to data collection to strengthen the methods of any outcome study. These steps will help make the data collection process more efficient, reduce potential errors in the data, and maintain a history of decisions made during data harvesting and coding.

The record of these steps is called a **coding handbook**. This handbook is a road map for the study. It contains the terminology, operational definitions, assigned numerical codes, and other procedures that are followed in the data harvesting. The coding handbook serves as a referral source for the clinician during data collection and interpretation. The following items are recommended for inclusion.

1. **Location of the variables.** The first step to coding data from patient records is finding the desired variables in the medical record. For example, if date of birth (DOB) is required, the location of the DOB in the clinic's patient record needs to be identified. Clinical settings organize their medical records differently. In hospital settings, DOB is often part of the admission information or is included in the identification card addressograph. In outpatient settings, there might be a designated space on the registration information that a patient completes, or a clinician might fill it in during the patient examination. It is helpful to record the typical locations for each variable as a reference source. This will help the clinician who is harvesting the data and is essential for training other clinicians to collect data in larger studies.

2. **Determine the format for recording each variable.** When a variable can be recorded in more than one way, the clinician needs to define the style that fits the needs of the study. For example, DOB can be recorded as numbers for the month, day, and year, or with the month spelled out, and with the year represented as two or four digits. ROM measurements can be recorded with either a 180- or 360-degree reference. Strength can be recorded in pounds, torque, or a combination of weight with repetition. Standardized tests with component scores, such as the FIM and the PEDI, can have the components recorded or just the total score. Before starting to collect data, the clinician will need to determine what level of detail is desired for each variable. Figure 10-3 is an example of a coding handbook.

3. **Convert text data into numerical codes.** One of the underlying rules about coding data is that all information should be converted into numerical data to facilitate statistical analysis. This is easy to do when the characteristic generates a number, such as degrees of range or minutes of activity. Nominal data, or data that label certain conditions or characteristics, need to have codes assigned to them. For example, in recording the sex of the patient, the choices are *male* and *female,* but text or letter abbreviations are not easily processed in electronic spreadsheets. Convert nominal labels to numerical codes by assigning a number to each of the possible conditions (e.g., female = 1, male = 2).

   One type of text data requires a random coding process: assigning case identification labels for patient identifiers. These labels are random codes that link the patient name or chart number with the coded data, and the list needs to be kept separate from the data in order to ensure confidentiality and objectivity. If there is a need to go back to the chart at a later time to retrieve or clarify data, the clinician will be able to break the code. When the study is complete, the identifying list should be destroyed.

4. **Create procedures for storing data.** Procedures for storing data are necessary so that data files are secure and recording forms are accountable. For small studies, portable file boxes, notebooks, or

---

A. Log = patient log #
    Enter pt log # i.e. (letter-#-date)

B. Clin # = Clinician Number
    Enter Clinician #

C. Diagnosis = Patient Diagnosis

1 = Lumbar sprain/strain	7 = Adhesive capsulitis	13 = Wrist sprain/strain
2 = s/p hand surgery	8 = Clavicle fracture	14 = s/p meniscal repair
3 = Vertebral fracture	9 = s/p CABG	15 = Elbow fx/dislocation
4 = Rotator cuff repair	10 = Knee problem	16 = Myofascial pain syndrome
5 = Femur fracture	11 = Talus fracture	17 = Muscle tear
6 = Chronic LBP	12 = Arthritis	18 = Ankle sinus tarsi
		19 = Combinations

D. # Goals = Total # of Goals at Initial Evaluation
    Enter # of Education, Impairment, Disability, and Handicap goals combined

E. (E) Goals = Total # of Education Goals at Initial Evaluation
    Enter # of Education goals (i.e. Home Exercise Program) or
    0 = No Education goal

F. (I) Goals = Total # of Impairment Goals at Initial Evaluation
    Enter # of Impairment goals (i.e. pain, edema, ROM) or
    0 = No Impairment goal

G. (D) Goals = Total # of Disability Goals at Initial Evaluation
    Enter # of Disability goals (i.e. ambulation, lifting) or
    0 = No Disability goal

Figure 10.3 Sample from a coding handbook. The letters and bold labels correspond to the spreadsheet columns.

file organizers that can be locked might be appropriate. Larger studies may require a dedicated locking file drawer. Computer files should be password-protected. If files have personal health information as defined by the Health Insurance Portability and Accountability Act, then procedures need to address maintenance of confidentiality and record security. In addition, consider where the study question, rationale, and related literature will be kept. Storing everything together will facilitate integration of the results with the literature and the reasons for conducting the study.

5. **Create accounting procedures.** When conducting a study in which several people are contributing to the data set, it is important to create procedures that track which records are entered by whom. These procedures should address how data recorders are identified, how to prevent one person from accidentally overwriting previously entered data, and how to ensure that coding reliability is maintained. If only one person is collecting data, it is still useful to have procedures for monitoring data recording forms. In the event that a procedure or coding decision changes, procedures will facilitate finding previously entered data.

6. **Keep an exception log.** An exception log is for recording decisions that are made when data do not conform to the rules. Decisions about how to use or discard these exceptions are recorded for future reference. Recording exceptions to data collection is helpful when interpreting the findings or when similar exceptions arise

again. When data are entered over weeks or months, it is easy to forget an unusual data coding decision. The exception log is a history of such decisions. Knowing how data have been treated or what data were omitted from the data set allows the clinician to interpret and report results of a study with greater fairness and caution. For example, suppose a patient previously treated for a chronic condition returns for a single consultative visit. If there were no prior coding options for a single consultation, a decision needs to be made about what to enter. The decision and rationale for the recording strategy would be listed in the exception journal for future reference. Then, when the next chart presents the same situation, the clinician will have a reference for how to proceed. The format of the journal can simply be a separate section of the coding handbook.

THE DATA RECORDING FORM

It is helpful to create a data recording form that includes all the variables in the study, all anticipated coding labels and their respective numerical codes, the method to indicate the chosen code for each case, and a place to make comments. Use one form for each chart reviewed to keep track of data and to reduce the potential for entering the wrong numerical code for transcribed data. Forms that allow the user to circle choices rather than fill in blanks will speed up the coding process and reduce misapplication of codes. Figures 10.4

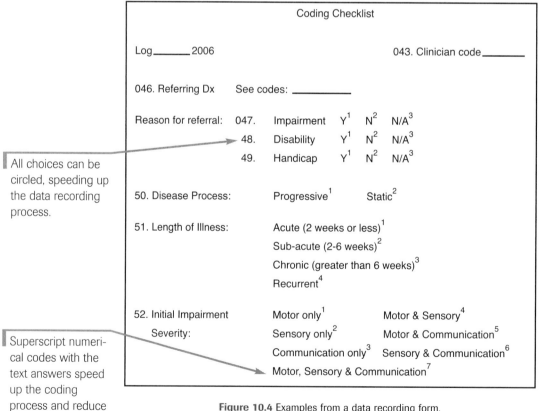

All choices can be circled, speeding up the data recording process.

Superscript numerical codes with the text answers speed up the coding process and reduce translation errors.

Figure 10.4 Examples from a data recording form.

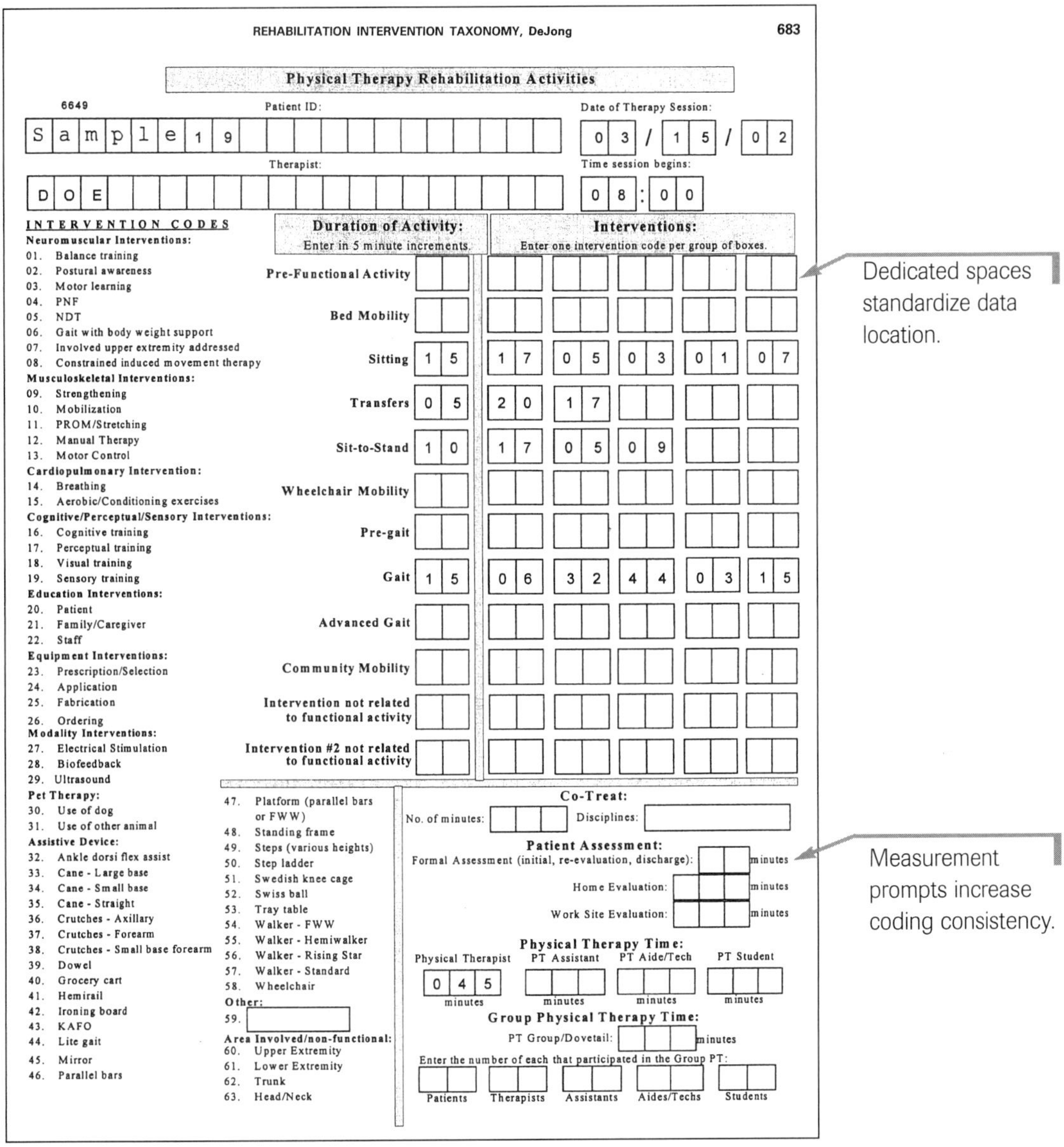

REHABILITATION INTERVENTION TAXONOMY, DeJong 683

Physical Therapy Rehabilitation Activities

6649 Patient ID: S a m p l e 1 9 Date of Therapy Session: 0 3 / 1 5 / 0 2

Therapist: D O E Time session begins: 0 8 : 0 0

INTERVENTION CODES

Neuromuscular Interventions:
01. Balance training
02. Postural awareness
03. Motor learning
04. PNF
05. NDT
06. Gait with body weight support
07. Involved upper extremity addressed
08. Constrained induced movement therapy

Musculoskeletal Interventions:
09. Strengthening
10. Mobilization
11. PROM/Stretching
12. Manual Therapy
13. Motor Control

Cardiopulmonary Intervention:
14. Breathing
15. Aerobic/Conditioning exercises

Cognitive/Perceptual/Sensory Interventions:
16. Cognitive training
17. Perceptual training
18. Visual training
19. Sensory training

Education Interventions:
20. Patient
21. Family/Caregiver
22. Staff

Equipment Interventions:
23. Prescription/Selection
24. Application
25. Fabrication
26. Ordering

Modality Interventions:
27. Electrical Stimulation
28. Biofeedback
29. Ultrasound

Pet Therapy:
30. Use of dog
31. Use of other animal

Assistive Device:
32. Ankle dorsi flex assist
33. Cane - Large base
34. Cane - Small base
35. Cane - Straight
36. Crutches - Axillary
37. Crutches - Forearm
38. Crutches - Small base forearm
39. Dowel
40. Grocery cart
41. Hemirail
42. Ironing board
43. KAFO
44. Lite gait
45. Mirror
46. Parallel bars
47. Platform (parallel bars or FWW)
48. Standing frame
49. Steps (various heights)
50. Step ladder
51. Swedish knee cage
52. Swiss ball
53. Tray table
54. Walker - FWW
55. Walker - Hemiwalker
56. Walker - Rising Star
57. Walker - Standard
58. Wheelchair

Other:
59. ____

Area Involved/non-functional:
60. Upper Extremity
61. Lower Extremity
62. Trunk
63. Head/Neck

	Duration of Activity: Enter in 5 minute increments.	Interventions: Enter one intervention code per group of boxes.					
Pre-Functional Activity							
Bed Mobility							
Sitting	15	17	05	03	01	07
Transfers	05	20	17				
Sit-to-Stand	10	17	05	09			
Wheelchair Mobility							
Pre-gait							
Gait	15	06	32	44	03	15
Advanced Gait							
Community Mobility							
Intervention not related to functional activity							
Intervention #2 not related to functional activity							

Co-Treat:
No. of minutes: ____ Disciplines: ____

Patient Assessment:
Formal Assessment (initial, re-evaluation, discharge): ____ minutes
Home Evaluation: ____ minutes
Work Site Evaluation: ____ minutes

Physical Therapy Time:
Physical Therapist 0 4 5 minutes; PT Assistant ____ minutes; PT Aide/Tech ____ minutes; PT Student ____ minutes

Group Physical Therapy Time:
PT Group/Dovetail: ____ minutes
Enter the number of each that participated in the Group PT:
Patients ____ Therapists ____ Assistants ____ Aides/Techs ____ Students ____

Figure 10.5 Example of a data collection form. (From DeJong, et al. [2004], p. 683.)

and 10.5 are examples of data collection forms. The former was used for a retrospective hospital chart review study, and the latter was used for a multicenter prospective study. Once the coding handbook and the data recording forms are complete, it is time to collect and enter the data.

PRACTICAL TIPS FOR ENTERING DATA INTO A SPREADSHEET

The following tips are geared toward clinicians who are performing their first outcome study. The assumption is that the data set will be entered into an electronic spreadsheet; however, the tips are just as applicable to paper-and-pencil spreadsheets and relational databases.

One Data Bit Per Cell

Only one number code should be entered in each cell of the spreadsheet. If a case has two diagnoses and both need to be coded, then two distinct columns need to be created. If two codes are put into a single cell, the spreadsheet software will not be able to recognize the information and may not include it in calculations.

Record the Smallest Unit of Measurement Possible

When deciding how to record a particular measurement, it is optimal to use the smallest measure that is reasonable for the study. For example, ROM measures should be recorded in specific degrees, not in ranges of 10-degree increments. Age can be recorded in years for adults, but it might be important to record age in months for toddlers if a difference of 3 months is relevant to the study.

Avoid Entering Transformed Data

Transformed data are data that have been manipulated, recoded, or collapsed into different values or labels prior to entry into the data set. Examples of transforming data include converting raw scores to percentages or pain scale measures to coded categories of "no pain," "mild pain," or "severe pain." When possible, data should be entered in their original measures. They can always be converted into less detailed groupings or summary units for a study, but if they are recorded only as transformed data, it will not be possible to go back and break the data down. For example, if a standardized test has three component parts, either the three section scores or the total score can be recorded. If the three section scores are recorded, they can be added to derive the total score, but if only the total score is recorded, it will not be possible to reconstruct the individual section scores without going back and reentering data.

Missing Data

When the information or measurement to put into a data cell is missing, it is helpful to have a code that indicates missing data. If the cell is empty, it is impossible to distinguish between cells that are accidentally skipped and cells for which the data are actually missing. It is best to create a missing data code that is uniquely different from the type of data that are typically entered in the column. For instance, by using a three-digit code (e.g., 999) for missing data in a column that records a two-digit code (e.g., year in school), the three-digit code will stand out during visual inspection of the data set.

Cleaning the Data

After all data have been entered from the data collection forms, it is important to review the quality of the data for missing data and typographical errors. One strategy for review is to print out the data set and look at the alignment of the numbers entered. If there are three-digit numbers where two-digit numbers should be and they are not missing-data codes, then recheck the data recording form. Another strategy is to run a frequency count on all of the variables and compare the results with the coding handbook.

If a code in the data set does not match the codes in the handbook, review the data collection form for that subject. A third strategy is to double-check the entry of data from randomly selected data collection forms. If there are many data, it is appropriate to conduct more than one type of data review to ensure that data are error-free (DePoy & Gitlin, 1998).

EXAMPLE OF A SIMPLE SPREADSHEET

This next section presents two stages of an evolving data set. In Figure 10.6, a simple spreadsheet includes some of the characteristics that could be harvested from patient documentation. The column headings identify the type of information, and the rows contain the findings for three cases.

In Figure 10.6, some of the patient information is entered as text, such as the patient names and the diagnoses. Because electronic spreadsheets do not recognize names as easily as they recognize numbers, these data should be coded with numbers. Enter the codes into the coding handbook so that the assigned numbers can be translated back into meaningful information.

In Figure 10.7, the initials and diagnoses have been converted to numerical labels. Now a spreadsheet program will be able to read the cells and provide frequency counts or other manipulations of the data.

SUMMARY

In order to analyze information about groups of patients, data about selected characteristics need to be organized into a data set. There are two formats for organizing data, flat files and relational databases. Flat files are two-dimensional spreadsheets that are appropriate for smaller, or simpler, data sets. Relational files are multiple spreadsheets linked by common identifiers and are better suited to larger, more complicated, data sets. A number of steps should be taken prior to harvesting data, including the development of a coding handbook and a data recording form, to increase the efficiency of data collection and reduce potential errors in the data set. Data should be recorded in their original rather than in a transformed state so that there is greater flexibility for analyzing and reporting them. Care should be taken before data are analyzed to ensure that the data set is as error-free as possible.

Patient Initials	Referral Source	Age	Referred Diagnosis	Date of Initial Evaluation	Payment Source
MM	1	35	Colles fracture	1/17/98	1
JB	2	45	carpal tunnel syndrome	1/21/98	2
PR	3	55	tennis elbow	1/21/98	3

Figure 10.6 Example of a simple data set.

Subject ID	Referral Source	Age	Diagnosis	Date of Initial Evaluation	Payment Source
079	1	35	1	1/17/98	1
234	2	45	2	1/21/98	2
561	3	55	3	1/21/98	3

Key: 1 = Colles fracture 2 = carpal tunnel 3 = tennis elbow.

Figure 10.7 Example of a revised data set.

References

DeJong G, et al (2004). Toward a taxonomy of rehabilitation interventions: Using an inductive approach to examine the "black box" of rehabilitation. Archives of Physical Medicine and Rehabilitation 85:678–686.

DePoy E & Gitlin LN (1998). Preparing data for analysis. In Introduction to Research: Understanding and Applying Multiple Strategies, pp. 235–245. Mosby, St. Louis.

Recommended Readings

Filemaker, Inc (1997-1999). Filemaker Pro 5: User's Guide. Santa Clara, CA.

Microsoft Corporation (1993-1994). User's Guide: Microsoft Excel.

Rothstein JM & Echternach JL (1993). Primer on measurement: An introductory guide to measurement issues. American Physical Therapy Association, Alexandria, VA.

Data Analysis

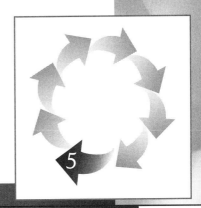

5

KEY TERMS

Descriptive statistics

Correlative statistics

Comparative statistics

Statistical significance

Clinical significance

Sampling bias

Procedure variability

Measurement bias

Historical bias

Experimental bias

CHAPTER OUTCOMES

➤ Define three levels of data analysis.

➤ Summarize the descriptive data for answering the sample outcome question.

➤ Identify common statistical processes according to the type of analysis they provide.

After data have been collected, coded, and entered into a spreadsheet, they need to be analyzed to answer the outcome question. This chapter describes steps to review data, the purpose of common statistical formulae, and typical sources of bias that should be evaluated when interpreting data analyses.

It is assumed that the clinician has introductory knowledge of research methodology and understands such processes as sampling, standardization of procedures, and basic applied statistics as well as such concepts as sampling bias, limitations, and generalizability. Examples of some of these concepts are provided but are not meant to be an exhaustive list of concerns. Research textbooks and statistical consultants can help to provide a more complete picture of data and assist the clinician in choosing the correct analyses. Statistical consultants are especially helpful with the use and interpretation of computerized statistics programs. In this chapter, the reader should focus on recognizing the responsibility for fair reporting and develop an awareness of potential consequences of incomplete or biased reporting. This chapter is not designed to teach statistics but rather to serve as a guide for how to organize statistics to answer a question. A list of recommended readings is provided at the end of the chapter.

A STRATEGY FOR READING THE DATA

Collecting data on an interesting question is like collecting pieces of a large jigsaw puzzle. Each piece of data is unique and belongs in a particular place. In the same way that the colors and shapes in a completed jigsaw puzzle are perused, it is important to peruse the completed data set. Some researchers refer to this perusal process as "letting the data speak" or "letting the data tell their story." These storytelling analogies are very helpful for reinforcing the idea that the strength of any conclusion is determined by the data that support it. Allowing the story or picture that the data naturally try to reveal adds a measure of protection against the biases about what an investigator hopes to find. During this process of data perusal, the clinician is looking for trends in the data, frequency and types of outliers in the data, and patterns of missing data, and is generally trying to get a sense of whether the quality of the data set reflects the expectations of the clinician.

Here are suggestions for perusing the data prior to analysis:

1. **Lay out all the data for viewing**. Print out the entire spreadsheet, and lay it out on a surface so that all the data are viewable.
2. **Look for missing data**. Look for blank fields where data are expected, and go back to the data recording sheets to check for accidental omissions or other reasons for missing or erroneous data.
3. **Look for the type of data expected**. Data can be entered incorrectly due to fatigue or if a key is accidentally hit twice. Wrong or duplicate characters can easily be mistyped or entered when a computer keyboard has a sticky key. For example, if age is entered in years, an entry of "700" instead of "70" might appear if the computer's zero key was accidentally hit twice or held down too long. Since a two-digit number is expected, a three-digit number will stand out in the column on the spreadsheet.
4. **Evaluate the data in each column for initial impressions**. Look for the range of the numbers, the variety or homogeneity within that

range, and whether the first impressions match what was expected. Sometimes during data collection, ideas are formed about what is collected. Stepping back from individual records and looking at the entire column of data may reinforce or minimize these first impressions.

5. **Write down the impressions from the data perusal**. Summarize what the data in each column appear to say. This is the foundation of the data's story. These initial impressions allow patterns to be seen in the data that may not have been anticipated. Later, when the data are run through statistical analyses, impressions can be confirmed or abandoned.

When these processes are completed, then data can be subject to formal analysis.

THE THREE LEVELS OF DATA ANALYSIS

There are three levels of analysis that can be applied to data: *descriptive* analysis, *correlative* or trend analysis, and *comparative* analysis. Descriptive analyses summarize patterns in the data. Correlative analyses describe how two variables are similar or relate to each other. Comparative analyses describe how two or more variables are different. Each level of analysis has a different purpose.

Descriptive analyses describe the distribution of data points for a variable or category. These analyses include such formulae as the sum, the mean, the mode, standard deviations, and frequency counts of nominal variables. In an outcome study, it is important to describe the *actual* sample of patients from whom the data are derived. While the hope is to collect data from a representative sample, the descriptive analyses will confirm if that actually occurs, or if there is a bias in the sample. For example, if a study includes patients between the ages of 40 and 60 years, the ideal data set would have patients representing all ages in the range and an average, or mean, age of 50 years. In reality, the sample may have been skewed, with 80% of the patients falling between 40 to 45 years old, resulting in an average age of 46 years. By describing the difference between who *could* have been included and who were *actually* included, both the literature and the data analyses can be more fairly interpreted in answering the outcome question. Descriptive statistics are generally performed on all the measured or recorded variables in a study.

Correlative, or trend, analyses describe the relationship of changes in one variable with changes in another variable. Examples of statistical formulae include the Pearson Product-Moment Correlation Coefficient (r), Intraclass Correlation Coefficients (ICCs), Spearman Rank Correlation Coefficients (r_s), and Point Biserial Coefficient (r_{pb}). It is often helpful to graph correlative data as scatter plots with measures of the two variables aligned along the X (horizontal) and Y (vertical) axes. (Fig. 11.1) A sloped line is calculated to represent the relationship of the two variables. The closer that line is to 45 degrees from the perpendicular axes, the stronger the correlation of the two variables. Numerically, correlation coefficients are reported as decimals ranging from 0 to 1, with 0 representing no correlation and 1 representing the perfect correlation.

Comparative analyses determine whether two or more groups of data are different or not and suggest cause-and-effect relationships between an inter-

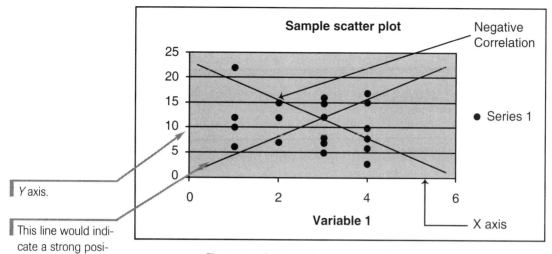

Figure 11.1 Anatomy of a scatter plot with correlation lines.

vention and an outcome. Comparative analyses include such formulae as t-tests, analysis of variance (ANOVA), Mann-Whitney U Tests, Wilcoxen Signed-Ranks Test, multiple analysis of variance (MANOVA), and analysis of co-variance (ANCOVA). The comparisons are often between pre- and post-test measures or between sample groups receiving different interventions.

The essence of comparative statistics is illustrated in Figure 11.2. This figure depicts the scattering of data collected from two groups of patients: group A received intervention A, and group B received intervention B. Comparative statistics determine the strength of the difference between the means of each group and the overall mean. If the group means are not different enough from each other, that is, if points A and B are not different enough from each other, then the comparison does not yield a statistical difference between the two interventions. If the means of the data from one or more groups are different enough from another group, then the comparison yields a statistical difference. The chance of a statistical difference is related to an interaction of the power or strength of an intervention to create a change in

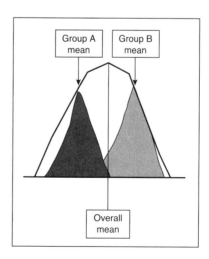

Figure 11.2 Illustration of the difference in means.

one group, the number of subjects in each group, the number of groups and interventions, and the range of measures recorded. The differences among statistical formulae are related to the type of data they were designed for, their ability to handle two or more than two groups, and the manner in which additional variables are controlled for.

STATISTICS FOR DATA ANALYSIS

The following list presents the types of statistical formulae that are typically used for describing, correlating, and comparing data in rehabilitation literature. Many of these formulae are also found as functions within spreadsheet and database software programs so that the tests can be performed on a data set without additional statistical software. The list includes only some of the more commonly used tests. They are provided for the reader to link the different levels of data analysis with the types of formulae associated with them. For more complete explanations of these and other statistical formulae, refer to a statistics textbook or the Internet.

Statistical formulae are organized according to the type of data they are designed for and the assumptions about the shape of the distribution of a variable in the population. The types of data include nominal, or labeled, characteristics (such as "male" and "female"), ordinal data (such as 5-point scales of "strongly agree" to 1 "strongly disagree"), interval data (such as temperature), and ratio data (such as age).

Parametric tests are based on the assumption that the population from which the study sample is drawn has a normal distribution. Parametric tests are typically applied to interval or ratio data. Nonparametric tests do not make assumptions about the distribution of the population from which the study sample is drawn and are typically applied to nominal and ordinal data.

Descriptive Statistics

Sum: The total resulting from adding a series of numbers.

Mean: The sum of observations divided by the total number of observations.

Mode: The most commonly occurring score.

Median: The middle score in a ranked distribution such that 50% of the scores fall above it, and 50% of the scores fall below it.

Range: The breadth of scores in a distribution equal to the difference between the highest and lowest scores.

Standard deviation: A calculation representing the spread of scores around the mean of those scores.

Frequency count: A total number of times that a variable code occurs; most often used with nominal variables.

Correlative Statistics for Parametric Data

Pearson Product-Moment Correlation Coefficient(r): Correlation statistic used to determine if the scores of two variables vary together.

Intraclass Correlation Coefficient (ICC): A reliability coefficient used to determine if the scores of two variables vary together and how closely those scores are matched.

Correlative Statistics for Nonparametric Data

Spearman Rank Correlation Coefficient: Similar to the Pearson *r*; for use with ordinal data.

Phi coefficient: Correlation of dichotomous variables in which each variable has only two values.

Point biserial correlation: Correlation of one dichotomous variable with one continuous variable.

Comparative Statistics for Parametric Data

Independent or unpaired t-test: Compares the means of two groups in which there are no repeated measures. The t-test assumes a normal distribution of the sample and random selection and assignment to groups.

Paired t-test: Compares the means of two repeated measures from the same sample group or from matched pairs of subjects.

Analysis of variance (one way): Compares the means of three or more groups on a single measure, or three or more repeated measures on the same group.

Analysis of variance (two way): Compares the means of two or more groups on two measures or repeated measures from two or more groups.

Multifactor analysis of variance: Compares three or more independent variables.

Comparative Statistics for Nonparametric Data

Mann-Whitney U Test: Compares the rank order of scores from two groups on an independent variable; the test can be used with unequal group sizes.

Wilcoxen Rank Sum Test: Similar to the Mann-Whitney U test; for samples of 30 or less.

Kruskal-Wallis One-Way Analysis of Variance by Ranks: Compares rank or ordinal data from three or more groups.

CHOOSING A STATISTIC

The choice of a formula to explore answers to a question is based on three factors.

1. What type of data will be analyzed in the question: nominal, ordinal, interval, or ratio measures.
2. Whether the intent is to show associations or differences in the data.
3. How many groups of data are included for a given analysis.

When choosing a statistical formula, it needs to meet all three factors. For example, suppose a clinician is trying to determine if there is a *difference* in the satisfaction levels of patients (rank or ordinal data) who receive treatments in the evening versus the morning (two groups). Given these factors, the choice of test would be the Mann-Whitney U Test, which is used to compare rank data from two groups. Decision trees can be quite useful in determining which statistic to choose. Figure 11.3 is an example of a decision tree Howell (2002) and Carlson et al. (2005) also provide three decision trees based on the type of data and the number of independent variables that are in a study.

INTERPRETING THE DATA

The investigating clinician is responsible for providing a fair and valid interpretation of the data. A fair interpretation of the data will recognize what has been found within the limits of the sample and the methodology. Explanations of why the interpretation or application of data is fair as well as what interpretations might be erroneous are important if the results will be shared with other parties.

Is The Question Answered?

A good starting point for data interpretation is to return to the original question, the rationale for studying it, and the strategies for how the data would be used. This review serves as a reminder of the original purpose for collecting the data and the changes in practice it was meant to support.

Second, it will be useful to review the Model for Rehabilitation Service Delivery described in Chapter 6. The model will provide a context for what had *hoped* to be included in the study or the types of procedures that were *anticipated*. Remember that, whereas the inclusion and exclusion criteria determined the subset of patients in the greater population that qualified for the study, the criteria are not a guarantee that the *actual* pool of participants will be equally represented in the sample.

Third, review and update the literature search to see if newer articles have been published since the study began. The results will need to be interpreted for the similarities or differences with existing studies. Confidence in the study's results is influenced by the strength of other findings available in the literature. Whether there is extensive literature to support what the study has found or no literature at all, the clinician is responsible for explaining what the results mean and whether they adequately answer the question.

Finally, determine whether the data analyses provide direction for improving service delivery. Remember, the purpose of outcomes research is to enhance practice by reducing the uncertainty about patient management, to improve efficiency and effectiveness of patient management, and to improve both patient and therapist satisfaction with the results of intervention. The study began with a question about practice and a rationale for studying it. Now the objective data should point to one of the three possible outcomes and strategies that were developed at the start of the study: a positive outcome, a negative outcome, or no difference in outcomes (see Chapter 8).

Statistical Versus Clinically Meaningful Results

Two different types of significance should be addressed when interpreting the results of data analysis. **Statistical significance** occurs when the data analysis results in a number that exceeds the level of chance. The criteria for exceeding the level of chance are specific to each formula and the degrees of freedom for the study. These criteria are organized in tables found at the end

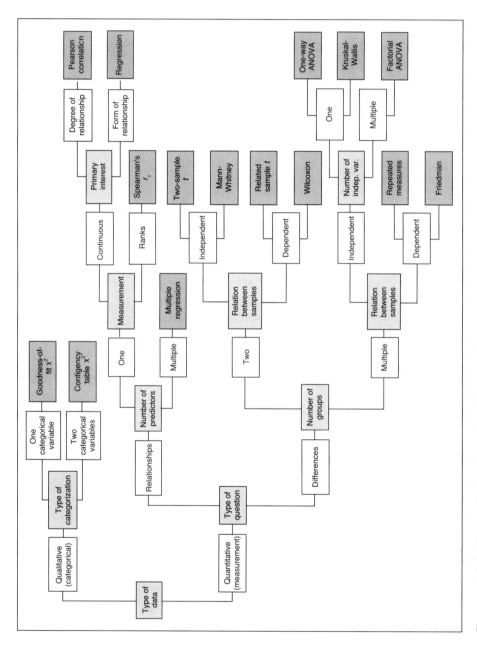

Figure 11.3 A decision tree for choosing statistical formulae. (Reproduced with permission from Howell DC [2005], from Howell, DC [2002]. Statistical Methods for Psychology [5th Edition]. Belmont, CA: Duxbury Press)

of any statistics textbook. If the analysis results in statistical significance, then the findings exceed the possibility that *chance alone* accounts for a trend or difference between groups.

It is important to remember that while the data analysis has yielded a statistical difference, it does not yield an absolute answer to the question. Generally, the question is directed at a broader group of patients than the sample actually measured. Consequently, the statistical significance applies to just the study's sample, which may or may not be a biased sample of the greater population of similar patients.

Clinical significance refers to whether the measured difference results in any useful changes. For example, if 30 subjects all gain 10 degrees of ROM following an intervention, a t-test might generate a *statistical* difference between pre- and post-test measures. If the additional 10 degrees does not allow the subjects to improve their level of functioning, then there may be little *clinical* significance to the findings. Conversely, if there is no statistical difference between pre- and post-test scores, but all of the subjects dramatically improve in their ability to perform activities of daily living skills, the change has clinical significance even though there is no statistical significance.

The types of significance are equally important. Interpretations of data from clinical studies should address both statistical and clinical significance in order to be fair and useful.

POTENTIAL LIMITATIONS TO A STUDY

Despite the best efforts to address potential limitations, clinical outcome studies that use retrospective chart review as a data source are riddled with limitations. Patients are not homogenous, charts have missing data, and sample sizes from a single clinician's practice may not be large enough to represent the true variations that exist within a diagnostic group. Some of these limitations exist even in the most carefully designed random controlled clinical trials. The responsibility of the investigator is to acknowledge the sources of bias or possible limitations and to interpret the strength of the results within the context of those limitations. This section reviews common sources of bias or methodological limitations.

Sampling Bias

Sampling bias exists when the actual sample of subjects has an imbalance of one or more characteristics and because of that imbalance, the group does not represent the typical subject profile that was defined. Two areas of common bias occur with age and sex distributions. For instance, the inclusion criteria may have included subjects from 60 to 80 years of age, but the actual recruitment may have resulted in subjects 60 to 67 years. In this case, the actual sample is biased toward the younger end of the recruitment range. Sex distribution is another characteristic that might contribute to sampling bias. If a study is open to all people, but only females are studied, then the sample is biased. The descriptions of the actual sample in the Model of Rehabilitation Service Delivery, as compared with the inputs that were not addressed, serve as reminders of the limitations of the actual data.

It is critical to appreciate the limitations of a sample before interpreting results. Smaller sample sizes will provide less generalization than larger samples, and samples from a single setting will be less generalizable than data representing multiple clinical settings. Biased samples are typical in clinical outcome studies as they are often samples of convenience. Patients recruited from a single practice setting may reflect a bias from the referral sources, geographic location, or the type of payment plans accepted. Charts that are reviewed retrospectively may be chosen based on completion of selected measures, and that may relate more to the diligence of the clinician than the inclusion criteria that the patients meet.

Procedure Variability

There are similar concerns to appreciate about the procedures that are documented. In a controlled research study, the interventions are applied to and documented in a standardized manner for all subjects in the treatment group. In contrast, the interventions coded for a retrospective outcomes study may not be standardized or applied to every patient included in the data set. In actual practice, clinical interventions are adjusted by a clinician for each patient based on a myriad of variables that are present at the moment of intervention. A sample may represent a wide variety of procedures or may have a bias toward one approach. Additionally, many interventions are provided and individualized without documentation of the details of those applications. Thus, charts included in retrospective studies may not reflect all of the specific interventions that were actually provided to all patients in the sample.

Measurement Bias

Measurement bias results from the *choice* of a measurement tool, from inherent errors associated with the *application* or *recording* of the measure, from limits of tool *construction* (e.g., selection of the items in a tool that create ceiling or floor effects), and from *variations in documentation* on the measure. For instance, in the approach to acute back pain, a description of examination processes in one practice might yield a broad array of tests and measures if the clinicians have been trained in a variety of approaches. On the other hand, if the clinicians are certified in a particular approach to back care, there may be a bias toward the examinations consistent with that certification process. Neither set of data is more useful than the other. It is the responsibility of the investigating clinician to interpret any results in light of the *actual* inputs and processes reflected in the data that might be unique to the measures used, recognizing their limitations when those processes are not representative of the true range of what *could* have been used.

Historical Bias

Historical bias occurs when an event happens outside of the patient care interaction that might influence some aspect of patient care service or outcomes. If medical records are reviewed from a period that overlaps the event, those records from the time before the event may yield different results than the records from after the event. Events that influence patient care occur all the time. Typical examples include changes in documentation requirements by third party payers, training of clinicians in a particular examination or intervention approach, administrative changes implemented by supervisory personnel, and even natural events (such as a blizzard) that influence the nature of problems with which patients present or their ability to access treatment.

Experimental Bias

Experimental bias occurs when either the participants or the investigators have expectations for outcomes because they know that they are being studied. These expectations may consciously or unconsciously sway their objectivity. In retrospective chart reviews, this is less of an issue because the patients and clinicians do not know that their charts will be selected, although bias can creep into the decisions about how items are coded. In facilities where random chart review occurs regularly, clinicians may also document differently if they expect their charts to be reviewed in the future.

Experimental bias can also influence the interpretation of the statistical results. When an outcome is expected, it is possible to "see" that outcome and not recognize other outcomes within the same data. The "blinders" of wishful thinking may thus influence what analyses are conducted, what results are reported, and what stories are missed or not explored.

SUMMARY

Data analysis comprises several levels. Raw data should be reviewed for their completeness and correctness as well as to visually identify trends in the data that may or may not have been expected. Descriptive statistics are used to summarize the characteristics of the sample and the measured attributes. Correlation statistics are used to calculate the strength of relationships between variables, and comparative statistics are used to compare two or more sample groups on one or more measured attributes. Statistical formulae are used to answer the outcomes question, but the clinician must decide whether the results are statistically and/or clinically meaningful. When interpreting data and statistical results, the investigator must be mindful of the possible limitations and biases that exist within the data, the methods, and the interpretation of results.

References

Carlson M, Protsman L, & Tomaka J (2005). Graphic organizers can facilitate selection of statistical tests: Part 1: Analysis of group differences. Journal of Physical Therapy Education 19(2):57–65.

Howell, DC (2002). Statistical Methods for Psychology, 5th ed. Duxbury Press: Belmont, CA.

Recommended Resources

Domholdt E (1993). Physical Therapy Research: Principles and Applications. WB Saunders: Philadelphia.

Polgar S & Thomas SA (2000). Introduction to Research in the Health Sciences. Churchill Livingstone: New York.

Portney LG & Watkins MP (1993). Foundations of Clinical Research: Applications to Practice. Appleton & Lange: Norwalk, CT.

Using and Sharing the Data

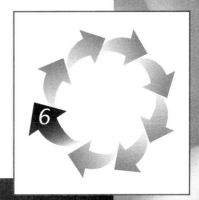

KEY TERMS

Outcomes orientation

Patient documentation

Service delivery

Staff development

Final report

Tailoring a report

Dissemination

CHAPTER OUTCOMES

➤ Describe a range of practice recommendations.

➤ Construct a summary report.

➤ Appreciate the different audiences for outcome data.

➤ Describe avenues for disseminating results.

This chapter describes the different ways outcome data can be applied to practice and provides a template for organizing a report. Considerations for tailoring a report and methods of dissemination are introduced.

Chapter 4, Consumers of Outcome Data, described various parties and their interest in outcomes studies. Any of the parties may have an interest in a study, whether or not it was originally intended for them. It is important to think about which stakeholders will have access to the report and the types of explanations they might need. Professional peers may already have insight into what they will want to know about. Patients might need lay interpretations of the data to avoid confusion or misinterpretation. For insurers, it is important to identify the types of clinical and business decisions to which the data might apply and to present both the application and its limitations. In all cases, think about the perspectives and needs of the audience, and adjust the presentation to represent the results and implications fairly.

CHANGING PATIENT CARE MANAGEMENT

The most immediate use of clinical outcomes data is their application to a clinician's daily decision-making processes. Data from a clinician's own patients should clarify what the clinician is doing well and what the clinician may want to change. The process of defining terminology and reviewing patient charts will illustrate where the clinician is consistent and where there is variability in practice. This self-awareness of personal practice patterns and levels of clinical effectiveness should influence how the very next patient is managed or how that care is documented.

If the data reflect the practices of more than one clinician, influencing practice patterns for a group of clinicians may be more challenging; however, the rewards of improved service are important. Remember that even small changes in patient care processes, such as documenting one new piece of information on every patient, may be harder to put into effect if some do not value the information as important. It will be the responsibility of the investigating clinician to educate others about the value of recommended changes.

POTENTIAL PRACTICE CHANGES RESULTING FROM OUTCOME STUDIES

The following descriptions are examples of the types of changes that might result from a simple outcomes study of a clinician's own practice. They reflect some of the more common types of changes that individuals make in clinical practice. The changes typically affect one of three areas: documentation, service delivery, and staff development.

Changes in Documentation Processes

Outcomes orientation of initial visit forms. Using an outcomes perspective in patient management means that the patient and the therapist agree on the same expected outcomes, and both understand how to measure or recognize when the outcome is achieved. Changes that clinicians have made as a result of implementing an outcomes orientation include:

- Documenting the patient's expectations for change or the patient's goals at the start of each examination.

- Reorganizing the layout of initial examination forms so that patient goals are documented early in the form.
- Documenting goals for functional activities rather than impairments.
- Providing a place in the documentation for the patient to sign or initial the goals, indicating that the patient knows and agrees with the expected outcomes of care.

Routine patient documentation. Studies of patient records often reveal less consistency in documentation patterns than clinicians expect. Studies of the frequency or timing of measurement recordings have resulted in such changes as:

- Identifying specific timelines for recording measurements.
- Standardizing the measurements recorded for every patient and/or the measures for patients with specific diagnoses.
- Standardizing the methods for recording information so that all clinicians use a single method or style.
- Clarifying processes for collecting specific types of patient measures (e.g., who gives a survey to the patient, which survey, and who collects it).

Use of standardized tests and measures. Studies of the types of tests and measures used to determine or record changes in patient status for selected diagnoses have resulted in such changes as:

- Building consensus among clinicians in a single setting on the types of measurements to be taken for selected diagnoses.
- Implementing standardized procedures or instruments for measuring patient status.
- Selecting different instruments as a result of exposure to current literature.

Changes in Service Delivery Processes

Service delivery processes refer to all the clinical and administrative activities experienced by a patient or that a business provides in order to manage a patient's episode of care.

Clinical processes. These refer specifically to a clinician's direct interactions with a patient and might include changes that result from both the review of the literature and/or the data gathering and analysis. Such changes might include:

- Increasing inclusion of the patient during interviews to determine meaningful outcomes.
- Using different measurement approaches or standardized tools.
- Selecting different interventions than those used prior to a study.

Administrative processes. Typical changes address what and how information is acquired, who collects and processes it, and how it might be used. Such changes might include:

- Reformatting intake forms to collect information that may not have been routinely collected before.
- Initiating surveys on quality-of-life or patient satisfaction.
- Clarifying clerical roles in distributing and collecting patient surveys.

- Converting to electronic documentation processes to facilitate internal data collection and analysis.
- Participating in examination processes that contribute data to national data sets.
- Instituting long-term follow-up procedures through surveys or phone calls.
- Initiating quality assurance or continuous quality improvement processes if none existed.

Cost and revenue analysis. Studies of costs and revenue are unique administrative outcomes related to providing services and might result in such changes as:

- Instituting alternative staff or patient scheduling patterns.
- Purchasing different types or quantities of products.
- Implementing patient follow-up procedures, particularly for canceled appointments.
- Expanding into niche practices that bridge services from clinical settings to community or wellness settings, based on needs identified by patients.

Staff Development Initiatives

Outcome studies on any aspect of the patient management process, including the types of examination processes used, the application frequency of selected interventions, or the consistency in documentation processes, can result in a variety of staff development initiatives. These include providing:

- Updated orientation processes for newly hired therapists.
- Continuing education for current staff to master selected standardized measures or documentation formats.
- Training programs to establish reliability in selected measurement tools.
- Training in quality assurance processes to ensure documentation consistency.
- Adoption or adaptation of clinical pathways.

POTENTIAL MISUSES OF OUTCOME DATA

The collection of outcome data is the basis of evidence-based improvements; however, there are misuses of data that can occur, intentionally or unintentionally. The investigating clinician should be aware of potential misuses and anticipate them in the preparation of presentations or reports. The consequences of misused data include basing decisions on data where type 1 or 2 errors exist (Rushton, 2000), basing policy and funding decisions on limited or misinterpreted data (Hebbeler, 2004), staff resistance or gaming to meet performance goals (Lilford, et al., 2004), and possible incorrect stigmatization of an institution or service (Lilford, et al., 2004). The following list of "red flags" is provided for the clinician to consider during the interpretation of the data.

- Basing major decisions on pilot data that might not yield the same conclusions if the sample size is increased.

- Basing major decisions on data from measures or classifications that have not been shown to be valid or reliable.
- Using outcomes data in isolation of the environment and processes in which it was collected.
- Failing to investigate the reasons for poor outcomes and lack of acknowledgment of other variables, including sampling bias, historical or confounding variables, that affect the outcomes.
- Failing to recognize limitations of the study's sample size or cohort, design or analysis of the data.
- Correlating patient clinical outcomes incorrectly with quality of care, as these are two different constructs.

Many changes can be implemented as a result of relatively simple outcome studies of personal practice patterns. The ability to spot trends in care, identify outliers, fill gaps in documentation, and reduce variability in processes justifies the efforts. This text focuses on studies of individual clinicians, but the processes apply equally well to groups of clinicians. Studies of multiple therapists in the same setting increase the opportunities to improve patient care logarithmically. Whether it is a study of individual or group practice patterns, data collection does not end with reading the results of the statistics table or comparing data from before and after a change in practice. All studies should end with a formal final report from which to build the next study so that the investigating clinician and others might understand what has been done. The next section addresses the construction of a final report and describes opportunities for disseminating the results.

CONSTRUCTING A FINAL REPORT

Formalizing the steps of a study into a written report is an important process, even if the clinician is the only person who will read it, because this is when some of the real insights occur. During this stage, the clinician must step back from the "micro" details of methodology to revisit the original question in the context of the Model for Rehabilitation Service Delivery. This "macro" view puts the study back into the broader context of the inputs, processes, and outcomes. The question, the variables studied, and the variables *not* studied need to be reconciled against the related literature, the data results, the new insights gained about practice, and the clinician's practical knowledge of service delivery. Writing the report requires careful articulation about the relationships among these variables; writing connects the logic between the problem that was first identified and the solutions that are implemented to improve practice.

Of all the stages of an outcomes study, this one should be the most fun! It presents itself as a puzzle or brainteaser and employs creative problem-solving to understand *why* the results occurred rather than *what* the results are. The choice to apply or not apply the results is based on an assessment of the validity and usefulness of the methods and the data. At this point, the clinician determines whether the study should shape changes in practice or whether to pause and collect more data. Finally, if there are practice changes that would be useful, the clinician identifies strategies that will work within his or her unique clinical setting and methods for measuring the outcomes of the changes that are implemented.

A Format for Reporting

The following outline will help to organize the written report. Each bullet indicates a new section, and the bolded phrases may serve well as headings.

- **The PICO or PIO Question.** Provide an introductory statement about the origin of the question or clinical problem, and then outline the original question in PICO/PIO format. The wording within the PICO format should read as a grammatically correct question. Avoid using fragments or statements that do not flow as a question, because this can be confusing to an outside reader (Table 12.1).
- **Rationale for the Study.** Explain the purpose of the study and how potential answers might influence clinical practice. This will help to focus the summary of the related literature and help others to understand why the study was important to conduct. Include references to support the need for the study or justification for potential actions that may be implemented based on the study's results.
- **The Bottom Line.** This is a brief statement that answers the question and identifies the action that will be taken as a result of the study. All elaborations of the answer and recommended actions follow in separate sections.
- **Methods.** This section should follow the same headings as most research papers. All of the procedures to create and analyze the data are described in enough detail to allow replication of the study.
  - **Sample.** Describe how the sample of records or patients in the data set was selected. Describe the inclusion and exclusion criteria, the number of records reviewed, and the number of records rejected.
  - **Statement of Institutional Review Board (IRB) Approval.** Studies conducted on data from patients treated by other clinicians and studies conducted with the intent to present or publish the results in public venues require the approval of an ethics or institutional review committee. This review is to ensure that no harm could come to any of the subjects as a result of inclusion in the data (Polgar & Thomas, 2000). Because this book focuses on retrospective chart reviews, the issues are more closely aligned with HIPAA regulations to ensure that the privacy of patient records and the rights of colleagues who created those records are maintained. Typically, studies of existing records that do not include

Table 12.1

Table of Sample PICO Questions	
PREFERRED FORMAT READS AS A QUESTION:	AVOID THIS FORMAT WITH FRAGMENTS:
P – For patients with type II diabetes I – does balance retraining C – as compared with hip strengthening O – increase standing time with eyes closed?	P – patients with type II diabetes I – balance retraining C – hip strengthening O – standing time with eyes closed

subject identification and personal health information may qualify for exempt status by the institutional review board, but the study still needs to be registered with a committee if the institution has one (Portney & Watkins, 2000a).

- **Chart Coding Processes.** Describe the coding processes for the inputs, processes, and outcomes measures. This is a step-by-step description of the variables studied in the question, their operational definitions, and their assigned codes. If any reliability testing occurred for the coding processes, describe that as well.

- **Data Analysis and Results.** This section of the report begins to answer the question. There are two ways that the section can be organized. Data can be presented following the statistical hierarchy of analyses; that is, descriptive, correlative, and comparative analyses are presented in that order. The data can also be organized by grouping analyses together for each variable or theme. If data were collected on more than one outcome, it may be helpful to group the descriptive summaries and the data analysis tables together for each outcome. Organizing the data by topic is recommended for outcomes studies because focus is maintained on components of the original question.

    Summary tables of the data should parallel narrative descriptions of the data. Just presenting the tables is not adequate; the clinician must explain the tables to orient the reader, provide an evaluation of the data as to their quality and how well they represent typical patients or practice patterns, and describe any exceptional situations that occurred during data collection that might influence their validity. The following are examples of tables that might be included.
  - **Sample demographics.** This includes descriptive statistics on variables of the actual sample, such as gender, age, and category or severity level of the diagnosis.
  - **Descriptive summary of the processes.** This includes frequency counts of coded processes or interventions from the records, if the study of processes is a central part of the PICO question.
  - **Descriptive summary of the outcomes measures.** This includes the most appropriate descriptive statistics (e.g., mean, mode, median, and/or standard deviation) on each outcome measure identified in the question.
  - **Statistics tables.** Include a table for each statistical calculation performed. Tables may present the results of correlations or comparisons of data. If multiple comparisons are made with the same statistic, such as a series of four comparisons, each using a t-test, present the four comparisons in a single table. It may even be possible to combine descriptive statistics with correlations or comparisons into a single table.
  - **Discussion.** This is the section where the clinician tries to make sense of it all. Organize the discussion by addressing the PICO question first. State whether there are any prior studies of the question or not. If there are, briefly summarize the findings of those studies. Avoid reporting on every study as a series of book reports. Use a grid of the literature to organize the summaries by topic. Include the articles that support key points and controversies, and avoid reporting on every article read (as there is

inevitably more read than is directly related to the question or the results).

It may be helpful to organize the remaining discussion according to the order of the PICO components. Describe the **P** (Patient) group studied. Identify the similarities or differences between the study sample and those in the published studies. Describe the **I** (Interventions) that were studied, the literature supporting the intervention activities, and whether the interventions have been studied before with the same methods of application. Do the same for any **C** (Comparison) intervention. Discuss the **O** (Outcomes) measured. Describe the different ways the interventions have been measured, what was found in the literature, and what was found in the study.

Discuss the methods and compromises made in the data collection process and interpret the strengths of the statistical results. Every discussion should acknowledge confounding variables (such as investigator bias or using a sample of convenience) that might temper the strength of the recommendations that are made.

- **Recommendations for Service Delivery.** Finally, present the recommendations that address the concerns outlined in the Rationale for the Study as well as any other discoveries identified along the way. This section is an elaboration of the "bottom line" earlier in the report. Identify the changes that should be implemented in a specific practice setting based on the original documentation formats, the data collection process, and the study's outcomes. The clinician should be specific to his/her practice setting as the data represent patients from that one setting only. In addition, the clinician should be reasonable. Twelve areas for improvement might be identified, but it is probably not possible to implement them all at once. The recommendations should be a blueprint for how to proceed, with changes, timelines, and the responsible parties identified. *Recommendations for practice changes should have measurable outcomes* so that improvements can be tracked. (These become the subject of the next outcome study, and the circle begins again.)

  If this sounds complicated, it is just a more detailed process of the same questions learned for elementary school reports. In summary, the report follows these questions:
- What is the question?
- Why was it important?
- What is known about it already?
- Who was studied?
- How were they studied?
- What was found?
- How does this study relate to other studies?
- How does this study clarify practice?
- Justify any recommendations for change.

Tailoring the Report for Different Audiences

When the initial draft is finished, consider tailoring the introduction and the discussion sections for the audiences who may read the report. An investigator can become so familiar with the concepts and processes in a study that providing the definitions or details needed by another reader might be over-looked. In addition, take care to explain the study limitations to reduce the risk of misinterpretation. Even if the investigating clinician is the only intended audience, it is important to tailor the report so that if or when a sub-sequent study is conducted following a change in practice, the clinician will have an accurate account of what the baseline situation was. Consider these conditions to determine the necessary level of detail or explanation.

A Study for Internal Use Only

It is perfectly legitimate to conduct an outcomes study that is used only for internal feedback and quality improvement. An outcome study is a photo-graph of practice at a single point in time. Just because a photograph is taken does not mean it should be used for public display. The investigating clini-cian needs to determine if the quality of the study and the data take a picture that is important enough to share with outsiders or if the data should only be used internally as a starting point to address practice issues.

When a single clinician conducts a study to evaluate practice patterns, the purpose is to reflect on practice and make improvements in that clini-cian's approach to patient care or documentation. Therefore, there needs to be enough detail in the final report so it is useful as a point of reference. The report should clearly outline the rationale for adopting or rejecting changes so that if a practice change is suggested in the future, the clinician has an evidence-based historical context from which to evaluate its merit. The report should also allow the clinician to replicate the study after making changes in practice to determine if the desired improvement in practice is achieved.

A Report That Others May Read

If an audience other than the investigating clinician will view the report, the amount of explanation provided is affected by who that audience is. If it is another clinician who shares some understanding of the language and processes studied, the amount of tailoring may be minimal. Keep in mind that even though clinicians in the same field may share an understanding of definitions and concepts, it is still necessary to provide a set of terms and operational definitions; these may differ among clinicians.

If the audience will be nonclinicians or clinicians with different clinical backgrounds, then more tailoring will be necessary. Outside audiences may not understand the exact nature of the problem or the processes nor how well this study represents the problem. The investigating clinician is the one who knows best how well the study represents the real clinical picture and is therefore the one who can best appreciate how confident anyone should be about the results. The tailoring should address the quality and consistency of the data, the types and numbers of exceptions made during data collection, and the level of evidence to support interpretations of the results. All limita-tions to the study should be carefully recognized and linked to any recom-mendations that are suggested.

When tailoring a report for others, think about how they might use the data or recommendations. They may be reading the study for different pur-poses. Clinicians may be concerned first and foremost with ways to serve patients better, whereas other readers may be more concerned with cost containment, or implications for other departments, or developing policy. The investigating clinician can have a strong impact on whether the results are interpreted in a fair and beneficial manner by anticipating the interpretations of the data for outside audiences. *The goal of tailoring a report for others is to support the recommendations fairly and to provide enough explanation to prevent the misuse of data or misinterpretation of recommendations.*

DISSEMINATION OF THE RESULTS

Conducting even a small outcomes study requires an investment of time and effort, and so much can be learned from the process. Methods of sharing what has been learned should be considered so that others might benefit from the efforts or be inspired to participate in reflective practice. The sharing may take place initially within the clinical setting in which the investigating clinician is working. Some of the insights that are identified along the way will probably yield recommendations that are useful to others. However, in addition to sharing the results internally, consider sharing them with other professional communities.

Dissemination of results refers to the processes of sharing the investigative experience, methods, results, and interpretations with larger audiences for the purposes of informing them and engaging in dialogue about the issues that have been studied. Each outcome study can be seen as a piece in a large jigsaw puzzle. Sharing the results enables a clinician to better understand where one study fits (or does not fit) with other pieces in the puzzle. Having opportunities to discuss the process and the results helps a clinician to recognize the strengths and limitations of the results and the implications that the study may have for others. Public discussion of results helps to keep a study in perspective and can also ignite new ideas about how to achieve the desired outcomes. Through this collegial dialogue, the study methodologies and interpretation of results are clarified, improved, or changed completely. It is from this rich dialogue with interested parties that the clinician grows as an investigator, that future studies become more directed, and that confidence increases for the skills of outcomes measurement.

Sharing the results with others may also inspire them to examine their own practice. They may learn of a new measurement tool or get an idea for how to examine their own service delivery. By sharing the results, the clinician will have improved his or her own practice and possibly that of other clinicians.

METHODS OF DISSEMINATION

There are several formats for sharing the results of a study. Each one serves different purposes and has slightly different benefits. Remember that if data are to be published for any public forum, the study methods should have the approval of an institutional review board.

Discussions

One of the simplest ways of sharing the outcomes research experience is through informal discussions with clinicians and researchers who are interested in the focus of the study. These discussions may occur in staff meetings, professional meetings, by telephone or email, or in writing, but the purposes are usually to clarify an issue or to hear another person's interpretation of something the study is addressing. These discussions can occur any time during the study, beginning with the identification of the problem through to interpretation of results. When outcomes studies are conducted as part of an ongoing quality improvement process, these types of discussions are common and do not require institutional review board approval.

Internal Reports

Clinicians and administrators within a clinical or institutional setting read internal reports. The investigating clinician may report to a clinical or business administrator or a governing board for the institution. In this type of report, the clinician would follow all of the same components discussed earlier, taking care to explain all jargon, concepts, methods, and limitations of the study so that statistical results are applied appropriately. Internal reports that are created for quality improvement processes typically do not need institutional review board approval as long as the studies were not conducted with the intent to publish the data for public review.

Poster Presentations

Poster presentations are formal presentations of the study in a graphic format on a large board. They are usually scheduled as a part of institutional, state, and national professional meetings. The process of preparing a poster gives the clinician an opportunity to identify the most important or exciting insights of the study to share with others. Because of the size limitations of posters, the clinician will need to whittle down the scope of the study to focus on specific points to share.

Generally, posters are available for viewing for several hours or days during a meeting. The clinician might be required to stand by the poster for a block of time in order to discuss the contents with others. These informal discussions provide opportunities to present the work verbally, to have the approach to the questions discussed, or to compare experiences with others who are looking at similar issues. Abstracts of posters are often published in monographs from the conference or in the sponsor's professional journal. Suggestions for designing posters address the readability of printed material, layout, materials, and use of illustrations (Portney & Craik, 1998; Portney & Watkins, 2000b). Applications to submit a poster may require an indication that the study received institutional review board approval.

Platform Presentations

Platform presentations are oral presentations to audiences that typically last 10 to 30 minutes. The conference committee hosting the presentations determines the time. Overheads, slides, or video clips to illustrate major points can accompany the presentation. The end of the presentation time is usually reserved for questions from the audience. This type of presentation is more formal than poster sessions. The title of the presentation, or the topic of a group of presentations, is often published in a meeting program, so anyone interested in the topic can attend. Presenting to a larger audience in a more formal manner can be daunting, but the formality of the process and the time limitations are helpful constraints when learning to identify which results from the study are important to share. Questions from the audience may seem challenging because the clinician is "on the spot." Be confident that as the one who conducted the study, the clinician is the expert, but the clinician needs to acknowledge that others may be experts in the methodology, inputs, processes, or outcomes. Responding to questions from the audience is part of a collegial dialogue that should help move the novice presenter past the feelings of *being tested* and onto the exhilarating realization that the study is actually something that others think is important. That realization is a confidence booster that inspires all investigators to continue doing research. Suggestions for organizing platform presentations address the timing, the layout and content of slides, and tips for verbal clarity (Portney & Craik, 1998; Portney & Watkins, 2000b). Applications to submit a platform presentation may also require an indication that the study received institutional review board approval.

Non–Peer-Reviewed Publications

Non–peer-reviewed publications in newspapers, magazines, trade journals, and electronic bulletin boards are not necessarily reviewed for scientific merit but rather for readership appeal. This form of publication can provide the clinician with practice in writing about the study, but other than acknowledgment for the efforts it may not gain the clinician much in the way of scholarly dialogue about the question raised. More often, these types of publications focus on reviewing published articles or literature reviews on a particular topic, not new, unpublished data. These types of publications are very useful for reporting about the experience of collecting data and the lessons learned along the way. Because these publications do not usually publish original data, institutional review board approval may not be required. However, if the clinician chooses to include original data, it is appropriate to indicate that the study was given institutional review board approval.

Peer-Reviewed Publications

Publications in peer-reviewed journals are considered the most rigorous form of dissemination and are most often focused on the presentation of original data. Articles presenting original data are required to indicate that institutional review board approval was received.

In the peer review process, the article is reviewed by the journal editor and by two or more colleagues with expertise in the content area. One of the reviewers will typically also have expertise in the type of research design used so that the appropriateness of the design, the statistics, and the interpretation of results can be reviewed. In a blind review, the reviewers are not given any identifying information about the manuscript's author so that objectivity is maximized. Manuscripts are often returned with suggestions for clarifications. Even the most published authors are asked to resubmit manuscripts, so the novice should not be put off by the request. This level of peer review should be seen as a written dialogue about the importance of the study's content, the rigor of the design for data collection and testing, and the clarity of the explanations.

When an article is published, the audience is endless and timeless. Depending on the readership of the journal and Internet availability, an international audience may be able to access the article at any time. In this way, the work is available to anyone with an interest in the topic, not just to those who happen to attend a poster or platform presentation at a particular meeting.

CONSIDER COLLABORATING

If the thought of disseminating a study publicly is overwhelming, consider collaborating with someone who is more comfortable with the process. Another clinician who has created a poster presentation or who has published in the area of interest may provide needed guidance and encouragement. There is greater comfort in company, and being accountable to another person is always helpful for meeting deadlines. By collaborating with someone, the clinician can share responsibility for the poster or article. Each person serves as a mutual reviewer for the clarity and accuracy of the work.

If collaboration is an option, it should start at the inception of the project. Then both parties can influence the methods and become knowledgeable in the related literature. Common etiquette is that persons who have primary responsibilities for the research design, implementation of the study, interpretation of the outcomes, and writing should be listed as authors or contributors in order of descending levels of contribution (Hoen, Walvoort, & Overbeke, 1998). Thus, in collaborating with someone to publish a study, expect to list the collaborators as authors if they have been instrumental in the execution of the study and the manuscript preparation.

When a clinician seeks advice about the process of constructing a poster or manuscript but conducts the study alone, colleagues review the work after the poster or manuscript has been drafted. At this level of assistance, the colleagues have had little to do with the processes of the study's design, interpretation, or writing; these people can be acknowledged at the end of an article but are not typically included as authors.

The benefits of sharing a study with others helps to clarify the clinician's own understanding of the work and helps others by adding to the knowledge base for practice. In this way, an outcome study will improve practice in the clinician's own setting but may have an even larger effect by improving practice in the settings of those clinicians who can read about the work.

SUMMARY

This chapter addressed two primary applications of the data. The first application is to inform the clinician's own practice to improve patient management and documentation. The second application is in the dissemination of findings to others who may have access to a report or who may benefit from the work. An outline of sections to include in a final report provides a method for organizing the study, from the question to the interpretation of how the data can or cannot be used to make clinical decisions. Both applications require careful reflection about the entire process of outcome measurement to determine how the data can enhance service delivery and an understanding that different audiences may use a report for different purposes. The clinician who shares a study with any other audience has the responsibilities of describing the study and interpreting the results with fairness and caution to minimize misapplication of the data.

References

Hebbeler K (2004). Uses and misuses of data on outcomes for young children with disabilities (draft). Early Childhood Outcomes Center, US Office of Special Education Programs, fpg.unc.edu/~ECO/pdfs/ECO_Outcomes_Uses.pdf

Hoen WP, Walvoort HC, Overbeke AJPM (1998). What are the factors determining authorship and the order of the authors' names? JAMA 280:217–218.

Lilford R, Mohammed MA, Spiegelhalter D, & Thomson R (2004). Use and misuse of process and outcome data in managing performance of acute medical care: Avoiding institutional stigma. The Lancet 363:1147–1154.

Polgar S & Thomas SA (2000). Presentation of health science research. In: Introduction to Research in the Health Sciences, 4th ed. Churchill Livingston, NY.

Portney LG & Craik R (1998). Sharing your research: Platform and poster presentations. Magazine of Physical Therapy, pp. 72–81.

Portney LG & Watkins MP (2000a). Ethical issues in clinical research. In: Foundations of Clinical Research: Applications to Practice, 2nd ed. Prentice Hall Health, Saddle River, NJ.

Portney LG & Watkins MP (2000b). Reporting the results of clinical research. In: Foundations of Clinical Research: Applications to Practice, 2nd ed. Prentice Hall Health, Saddle River, NJ.

Rushton L (2000). Reporting of occupational and environmental research: Use and misuse of statistical and epidemiological methods. Occupational and Environmental Medicine 57:1–9.

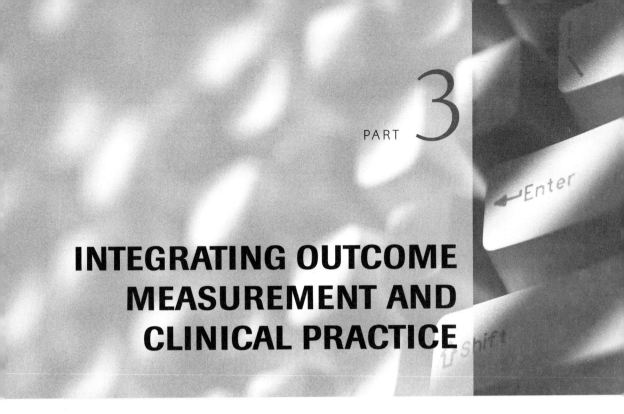

## PART 3

INTEGRATING OUTCOME MEASUREMENT AND CLINICAL PRACTICE

Part 1 of this text presented foundational information about using an outcomes perspective, domains of measurement, and models to help organize aspects of patient management. Part 2 provided direction about conducting a retrospective study of patient charts from a clinician's own practice as a method for reflection and evidence-based practice improvement. Part 3 addresses the larger systems view of service delivery and how outcomes measurement and management can be used as ongoing processes.

When thinking about implementing changes in practice or conducting outcomes studies that include other clinicians, there are additional factors that should be considered. Of the many benefits of conducting larger-scale studies, the most obvious is that the results will better reflect true practice. On the other hand, as studies grow to encompass other participants, someone needs to be leading the way. The study manager needs to be aware of potential costs, concerns of staff, and the responsibilities involved with leading a group through the reflection process. Part 3 introduces the issues that a study manager should consider before conducting larger scale studies and methods of integrating outcomes measurement with quality improvement processes based on these larger studies.

Considerations for Conducting Outcome Studies

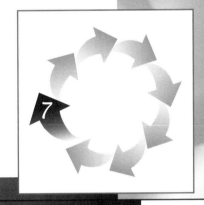

## 13

KEY TERMS

Project manager

Communication

Education

Morale

Consensus

Project costs

CHAPTER OUTCOMES

➤ Describe the responsibilities of an outcomes manager.

➤ Describe aspects of staff preparation.

➤ Describe the costs associated with outcome studies.

➤ Identify strategies to enhance success.

Conducting outcomes studies can seem like a daunting process to the individual clinician. Even the simplest studies require careful thought, diligence, and time to identify the question, collect the data, and interpret and use the results. The efforts are not immune to Murphy's Law ("if anything can go wrong, it will"), so that missing data, computer viruses, and hindsight about what could have been collected can unravel the nerves of the most ardent data collectors and committed clinicians. Nevertheless, the only way to move the quality and accountability of physical therapy services forward is through the thoughtful process of comparing objective evidence collected before, during, and after changes in practice patterns. Once a study is completed, the next study seems less daunting.

Until now, this book has dealt with evaluating the outcomes of a single clinician. When outcome studies expand to include data generated by multiple clinicians, there are factors that need to be considered to maximize success. This chapter will review the logistics of conducting a retrospective study on multiple therapists.

OUTCOME ADDICTION

The insights realized about practice and documentation patterns can be quite powerful for the individual clinician, causing the sanest person to charge into a staff meeting with mandates to implement a list of changes. This transition from the reflective clinician to the militant outcomes guru sometimes occurs with data from a small pilot study or a sample from a single diagnostic group. The data hardly represent the full breadth of the clinician's practice; however, the lessons learned from the process of conducting the study leave such strong impressions that the clinician feels compelled to share them. Such is the emotional reaction that completing a study can have.

The assumptions and memories about how service is delivered and what is recorded prior to an outcomes study are often challenged by the actual data that are available to harvest. Sometimes there is pride (and relief) in the strength of the documentation process because a data set was easy to assemble or because the results confirm the expected outcome. Sometimes the clinician is frustrated by the data harvesting process, embarrassed by the inconsistencies in the data, or surprised by results that conflict with expectations. Regardless of whether the clinician's assumptions about practice and documentation are supported or whether the results lead to significant changes in practice behaviors, there is a strong realization that conducting the study was the only way to see the situation objectively. And the clinician is hooked!

To avoid misapplication of a study's results and to temper the desire to recruit other clinicians to accept a study's recommendations, consider the following issues.

Pilot Data May Not Fairly Represent Practice

If the first study conducted has a small sample size, then the data may not represent the true variability that might be present in patients or in the documentation on patients. Any recommendations based on small sample sizes should focus on increasing the consistency of documentation or standardization of procedures but should be conservative when recommending changes in patient management.

Biases in sampling are common during pilot studies. Multiple charts may be reviewed, but only those with adequate documentation are selected into the data set. The charts that were passed over are unrepresented in the data. Had those charts been included, the results and recommendations might look very different.

In the case of a small sample size, the clinician has two options. The first, highly recommended, option is to add more subjects to the study and rerun the statistics. If the original results hold up, then the clinician's confidence in the results can increase. Second, the clinician should identify the most variable aspects of documentation that might affect the results and implement changes to decrease variability. Another pilot study should then be conducted to see if the expected reduction in variability occurred.

One Clinician May Not Reflect Other Clinicians in a Practice

The data from one clinician tell only the story of that one clinician. Although there may be an assumption that the same inconsistencies in documentation might be apparent in other clinicians' charts, that assumption needs to be verified with data from their charts. Be careful not to generalize recommendations to all staff when the data represent only a single person. In this case, the clinician should present the results to the staff, being clear that this is a study of one person. Then there are two options. Individual therapists can be encouraged to conduct the same study, or a single group study can be recommended. The latter may be more threatening, as everyone's bad habits will be hung out for public viewing.

Learning About Outcome Studies Takes Time

The reflective practitioner who accepts the challenge of conducting a study may not feel comfortable with exposing documentation habits, but the idea of improving practice is more compelling and spurs a clinician past any personal reluctance. This personal commitment to increasing accountability in practice is a strong motivator that may not be a priority for others in the same clinical practice setting. The clinician who has completed an outcome study needs to honor the variations in comfort that others feel about objectively measuring their practice patterns. Imposing an outcome study on someone with minimal comfort can turn a well-meaning activity into a threatening one.

The process of learning outcome measurement takes time. The investigating clinician should remember that the steps learned during each phase of the project occurred as a gradual process, so there was a long lead time to arrive at the current level of understanding. The recommendations at the end of a study are just part of the benefits realized. The clinician must be careful to appreciate the learning curve when trying to extol the virtues of outcome data. Other clinicians in the same setting will not have invested the time nor have the same knowledge of conceptual frameworks, terminology, or processes. Attempts to make changes or to recruit others to open their charts for self-examination may be met with resistance. Therefore, a deliberate process of enculturation and education should be considered to bring others up to speed and to gain cooperation.

If multiple pilot studies on the same issue or increasing the sample size yields consistent results and staff appear interested in the process that has been role modeled, then the environment might just be ready for a multi-clinician study. If this is the case, a project manager should be identified who will oversee the organization of the study's processes.

PROJECT MANAGER RESPONSIBILITIES

Commitment and Communication

The project manager should possess the energy, commitment, and basic knowledge to conduct an outcomes study. The manager should be able to design a study, or know when to collaborate with a consultant, and be knowledgeable about the tools used to gather and enter data. The manager may be responsible for training appropriate staff in their roles and for organizing the process of data collection and report generation. It is helpful if the project manager is knowledgable about statistics and data analysis but, if not, it is more important that the manager be able to collaborate with a statistician effectively. Finally, the manager should be an excellent communicator and motivator. This person will be responsible for educating staff about the goals, procedures, and benefits of a study; for giving feedback and encouragement along the way about data acquisition; and for describing the results and their meaning for the practice. Successful communication with peers is essential for keeping staff interested and committed to contributing accurate and complete data.

Identifying a Question

A project manager can identify many questions to study, but to increase the participation of multiple clinicians, it may be wise to ask them about perceived needs. The project manager should be prepared to get anything from no responses to a barrage of responses. If there are no responses from the clinicians, the project manager is free to suggest one that might have broad appeal. A barrage of responses may require some tact to identify one study without alienating other clinicians.

One solution to an enthusiastic response to what to study is to develop a series or list of questions. The project manager presents a priority order for questions, which includes assessment of the related costs and potential benefits to the practice. The simplicity of starting with one question allows for data collection procedures to be kept simple. The priority order of subsequent questions allows the project manager and other members of the team to see when other interests will be addressed. As information from the first study can influence the direction of later investigations, the priority list becomes a working document that is reorganized according to the information and experience gathered from all previous studies.

Time and Task Management

The project manager should be organized and have effective time management skills. This person will be tracking data collection from several sources and possibly maintaining clinical responsibilities. The ability to manage multiple processes simultaneously and keep everyone positive about the experience will be important to the success of the study.

Institutional Review Board Preparation

In settings that have institutional review board (IRB) procedures, the manager may be responsible for preparing the documents and responding to an IRB committee's request for clarification. The manager should be familiar with the types of studies that require review and understand what a committee is looking for in the application. The manager may need to submit an informed consent form as part of an IRB application that is understandable by the patients whose records may be used for data collection. In settings where there are no formal IRBs, an informed consent form that follows the federal guidelines should still be provided to patients so that charts can be used. Additionally, it would be in the clinical setting's best interest to create a committee to review a study's protocol. One or more committee members should be familiar with federal requirements; such individuals may be contacted at any university or medical setting in which research is conducted.

Education and Morale Management

The project manager is responsible for staff training and morale. Participants may be solicited as volunteers, or they may be assigned to participate. Volunteers may have a higher level of interest in the project, comfort with research activities, and appreciation for the standardization of processes that are part of research methodologies. When training volunteers, a manager is educating people who may already believe that there is merit to conducting the study.

Clinicians who are assigned to assist in an outcome study may present the manager with some obstacles to full participation. One obstacle is that of perceived additional workload. Current documentation processes are quite involved and time-consuming. When clinicians are assigned to participate in additional chart review activities or documentation processes, the potential for no or partial compliance with documentation increases. The project manager needs to ensure that all staff members understand why data are being collected and how they will be used to support the integrity of the study's procedures. Describing the big picture and where the different steps of a study are within that big picture helps staff to understand why a study is being conducted and where it will lead. Just as a clinician and patient must have a good understanding of the outcome of intervention, so must the manager and staff have a good understanding of the goal in order to participate fully in the process.

Preparation of the Final Report

The project manager will translate all of the processes and recommendations into a report. The components of the report were described in Chapter 12. This section addresses the option of organizing members to contribute to the report.

If others have been heavily involved in the outcome study, it may be desirable to invite them to participate in writing or editing selected sections. The project manager will need to set dates, clarify the topics or sections to be written, identify the style guidelines that writers should use, and facilitate the collection of the drafted sections. By organizing the tasks before they are assigned, the project manager will be able to monitor the completion of the report.

Care should be taken to edit the assorted components that others contribute. The final report should read as though it had a single author. Redundant sections are not unusual, as one clinician may not have known that another clinician described the same issue. Terminology may be applied differently and should be edited for consistency. Even formatting of headings and tables may take on different styles, and all should be aligned along one set of standards. After a final draft is completed, provide everyone who has had significant roles in the study with a chance to edit or clarify the report before printing and disseminating it.

STAFF PREPARATION

There is an old saying: "Garbage in, garbage out." In outcome studies, the results are only as good as the data collected, and their quality depends on the clinicians who document the data. When multiple clinicians are involved in a study, larger data sets can be developed more quickly, but there are also more opportunities for data to be compromised. This section will review some of the variables that can affect the results of a multiclinician outcome study.

Consensus on the Need for Studying Outcomes

Consensus begins with developing agreement among staff that some evaluation of practice needs to occur. On the surface, it may seem like an easy idea to agree with; after all, most clinicians want to deliver the best service possible. In fact, however, collecting outcome data can be perceived as threatening to individual clinicians for several reasons.

It is threatening because of the relative value that is placed on a process or topic that is chosen for study. Just by being studied, a process is identified as important to understand more thoroughly. Clinicians who do not participate in or use that process may feel left out of something important, or they may feel that the processes with which they are involved are less worthy of study. Convincing staff about the merits of a study can be handled by developing a long-term plan that defines the purpose and steps of collecting outcome data and the opportunities for contribution by staff along the way.

A clinician may disagree with the choice of outcome to be studied and believe strongly that a different outcome study would better serve the practice. In this case, discussion of the reasoning for each of the proposed studies may help staff to understand why one study is selected over another. The discussion should include the logistics required to execute each study: the number of staff members involved, the number patients needed to create a data set, the time in which the data can realistically be collected and, critically, the immediate problems that will be resolved as a result of the study. By describing the merits and expected outcomes of a variety of studies, it may be possible to compose a long-term plan for outcomes research that addresses everyone's interests.

Consensus on the need for studying outcomes is easier to obtain in settings where there is a trust and respect among the staff. When clinicians value the contributions that everyone makes toward a practice, singling out one question to study is less likely to be interpreted as an inflated importance of that question or as a minimizing of the questions that are not studied.

Consensus on the Use of Data

Clinicians may be threatened if they think data will be used to influence decisions about employment status, bonus awards, promotion opportunities, or other personal aspects of professional advancement. For example, outcomes studies that code who the clinician is for each patient may be useful for comparing how a master clinician practices in comparison with a novice clinician. This type of study, however, may spur concerns that the data will be used to influence performance reviews and employment status. Staff members who feel threatened in this area need clear and overt reassurance that performance review is based on a broad constellation of skills, not the outcome of a single statistical finding. Additionally, if the purpose of an outcome study is to identify evidence of best practice, then staff will need reassurance that the findings will lead to staff development to promote excellence in all rather than selective reward or, worse yet, layoff of anyone interpreted as less effective.

The Value of Identifying Best Practice Patterns

Staff may perceive that an outcome study will promote standardization of interventions, resulting in a loss of clinician creativity and individualization for the patient. In this case, staff may need to be reassured that there will always be room for creative problem-solving in the application of interventions. On the other hand, the notion that standardization of measures or interventions is perceived as a negative trend in practice also needs to be reversed. Much of the variety in a clinician's approach and the constant hunting for new interventions may be a direct result of the lack of available evidence to support what works. If there were evidence to show that one intervention approach is more efficient and effective, most clinicians would conform to that norm, knowing that it was the appropriate intervention to provide. In fact, evidence-based protocols and clinical pathways for the management of such diagnoses as stroke, total knee and hip replacement, and hip fracture have been shown to decrease hospital stays, improve long-term outcomes, reduce costs, and improve care (Baker, et al., 1998; Kim, et al., 2003; Koval, et al., 2004; Thomas, 2003; Wee, et al., 2000).

The Impact on Documentation Time

Clinicians may fear that the collection of outcome data will become an additional burden during documentation. When schedules are very tight and documentation requirements are already lengthy, this stands as one of the greatest obstacles to practicing clinicians. Documentation time and methods should be given careful consideration when developing methods for capturing data.

For retrospective chart reviews, the project manager needs to determine how many clinicians are involved in data harvesting. One option is that the project manager collect the data from other clinicians' charts. In this case, the clinicians will not experience any additional documentation time. At the other extreme, every clinician might be required to submit data from a group of charts. Although this shares the work and speeds up data collection, the introduction of multiple coders requires more training to ensure coding reliability and more consensus-building to ensure that everyone adheres to the methodology. Typically, data harvesting falls to a few clinicians who express an interest in helping. Volunteers bring a measure of commitment to the study, and they are more apt to perceive the additional work as a learning opportunity. The point is that when more clinicians are involved in data collection, there are greater risks to coding reliability, but when fewer clinicians are involved, there is less transparency to a study, which may cause greater suspicion by clinicians whose charts are included for data harvesting. Clear and frequent communication is an important strategy for minimizing perceptions of secrecy.

In the case where a pilot study recommends documentation changes so that future retrospective studies have specific data more available, careful thought should be given as to how to collect the additional information. Devising separate forms may be easier for the project manager, but such forms may be more cumbersome and redundant for the clinicians. Data capture procedures should be as time-efficient and integrated into the current documentation processes as possible. Data capture may be achieved by adding a few items to an already standardized intake form, standardizing answers to circle as clinicians complete a form already used by the practice, or by providing a pre-visit questionnaire to a patient at check-in so that time with the clinician is not compromised. Conducting an outcomes study will require additional work by everyone, but communicating the desire to incorporate that work into the natural flow of practice and respecting clinician time will go a long way to improving data collection compliance.

Documentation Changes

Clinicians may be reluctant to use standardized evaluations or note-writing formats (Russek, et al., 1997), but outcome studies require that very specific types of information be collected and documented in the same way by each participating clinician. The use of standardized measurement tools may also require training for users to become reliable in scoring the instrument. There are some strategies that can enhance proper and complete documentation.

When designing an outcome study, identify the variables of interest as well as where the data are already collected. Capturing data already documented as part of the medical record decreases the perception of added burden. Because the clinicians are already recording this information, it may only be necessary to standardize the way in which items are recorded.

For data that have not been routinely collected but that will be added to routine documentation for use in future studies, it helps to devise a documentation format that is easy to understand, easy to complete, and easy to access. Ease of understanding relates to the use of definitions that are clear to everyone, thus reducing ambiguity about how to label or code a patient response. Arranging answers that can be circled or listing items with boxes to check off decreases variation in the types of answers documented and increases the speed with which items can be completed. Finally, the format for data collection should be easy to access. If a form or measurement tool is added to documentation, it is important to identify a process that gets the form to every clinician who needs it. This may be as simple as keeping a pile of forms available in an identified location or having clerical staff insert the form into patient charts. If the items that need to be documented are inconveniently located, they will be forgotten during the rush of the day's activities, resulting in missing data.

Staff Reliability for Coding Data

After operational definitions have been identified and the methods for coding patient variables are accepted, staff must be trained to establish an acceptable level of reliability. Inter-rater reliability refers to the ability of those coding data to rate the same situation, characteristic, or quality the same way. The project manager will need to ensure that codes are applied the same way and that coding exceptions are communicated to all involved in data harvesting. When multiple clinicians are involved, it is not likely that they will all perform chart reviews at the same time, in the same location, and in the same manner. Establishing methods of communication to update everyone will assist with maintaining coding reliability.

Staff Reliability for Patient Documentation

The project manager will want to ensure that all data contributors are applying tests and measures in the same way. Inter-test reliability refers to the ability to administer a test on two separate occasions and produce the same results, given that nothing else has changed. The conditions for administration and the methods of documenting the results must be the same. As new people begin working at a facility, they will need to know what parts of a study are dependent on their actions and then receive training in order to perform them accurately. Staff members who have been contributing data should undergo periodic reliability tests to ensure that the expected administration and documentation standards are being maintained.

Appreciation of Everyone's Contributions

The success of a study will be increased if everyone in a clinical setting understands and supports the types of work that will be needed from its members. Those who use more time for data collection and analysis must understand that others may be supporting the effort by accepting heavier patient loads or other administrative responsibilities. Those responsible for information coding, including students and volunteers, must understand the importance of complete and accurate data. When all members are committed to the investigation, the accuracy and efficiency of data collection can be maximized. The project manager plays an important role by publicly acknowledging everyone's contributions on a regular basis.

THE COSTS OF STUDYING OUTCOMES

There are a variety of costs associated with performing outcome studies. The more obvious costs might include the purchase of consultative services, computer hardware and software, the salary to support a person to do data entry, the purchase of assessment kits/forms, and possibly membership into a commercial data set. Some of the less obvious costs are important to recognize. This section will review some of the hidden costs of conducting outcomes studies.

Time

Remember the concept: "Time is money." Indeed, conducting outcomes studies requires an investment of time. Time is needed to prepare for and learn about the processes that are needed. Time is needed to meet with staff about the plans and to train those will be contributing or coding data. Clinicians need time to find and read the literature related to the question. They will need to complete additional data fields or forms, and someone will need to spend time to input, analyze, and finally report on the data. If a staff member is freed from patient care to oversee and participate in data collection and management, that person may be treating fewer patients. Somehow, the time spent by clinicians participating in or organizing outcome study activities will need to be funded.

Requiring additional staff meetings for training may mean that clinicians need to treat more patients simultaneously to free up time. Using documentation processes that are lengthier than current practices may mean that therapists have more administrative work related to their current patient load. While neither is necessarily problematic, these scheduling patterns may be different from the way everyone has preferred to provide services. Alternative scheduling, more administrative time, and training time to implement new procedures may require financial support.

Training and Supplies

If a standardized test or measure is selected that requires training to ensure reliability, staff will need to be trained in its administration. This might require hiring a certified trainer, sending staff to a certification course, or paying for a training video kit that comes with reliability scoring processes. In these examples, the first two options are bound to be more expensive than the third, but all three will require an investment of staff time on top of the training costs.

Some tests must be purchased for use. Administration kits, scoring manuals, and blank scoring forms may have copyright protection so that when forms run low, additional forms need to be purchased. This supply cost will vary depending on the type of measurement tool chosen, the number of patients who will use them, and the number of times a tool is administered on a patient for data collection. If the patient will be reexamined on several occasions, for instance at the initial visit, at discharge, and 3 months after discharge, then more copies of a tool will be needed to complete the documentation. These proprietary instruments have costs that need to be factored into the choice of tests and the frequency of administration.

Number of Charts to Review

The primary considerations about the number of charts reviewed for a data set are their availability and the format of the data. Depending on the specialization of the practice, the frequency with which a practice admits patients with the same diagnosis will vary. Diagnostic categories with high frequencies allow for more rapid data collection on that diagnosis than diagnostic categories with low frequencies. The outcomes manager will need to estimate the data collection period based on typical frequencies of patient diagnoses.

Shorter data collection periods have the advantages of keeping the staff interested and keeping data documentation skills at a reliable level. They have the disadvantage of compressing the two needs of managing a caseload of patients while completing the retrospective chart reviews. The intensity and pace of this compression can be kept up for a short time before clinician interest starts to decline. One way to relieve the compression of responsibilities on current staff is to bring in additional temporary staff to assist with patient care when data coding is under way.

Longer data harvesting periods should be planned for patients with lower frequencies of referral. Unless the clinic has an electronic search method for identifying patient charts that fit the inclusion criteria, a manual search of records may need to occur. With lower frequencies of occurrence for a specific diagnosis, many more charts will need to be reviewed to find the charts of interest.

Another disadvantage to long data collection periods is the increased difficulty in keeping everyone's interest in and commitment to the process. One strategy to enhance data collection on patients with less frequently occurring diagnoses would be to collaborate with another practice that may be seeing similar patients. Increasing the potential pool of eligible patients may successfully shorten the data collection period. Just be aware that collaboration among sites increases the time needed to ensure inter-site reliability.

Membership Fees

Businesses provide electronic documentation processes and support outcomes studies. There are currently two organizations that have well-established mechanisms for collecting data from member affiliates. These are the Focus on Therapeutic Outcomes, Inc. (FOTO), for outpatient orthopedic data, and the Uniform Data System for Medical Rehabilitation, which collects pediatric and adult rehabilitation data. Both these organizations offer important benefits that are included in the cost of membership. They provide training and ongoing support to their members for their data collection processes. Both take data and provide a profile that describes how a patient compares with others with similar issues and how the clinic looks relative to similar clinics in the data set. One disadvantage of becoming a member of a specific outcome measurement group is that a clinician may have outcome interests that are not the same as those of the company. The clinician's specific questions may never be answered by the nature of data that is collected or may be available only for additional fees. Nevertheless, the types of data and reports that are provided have been found useful by many clinical settings and help the novice understand that outcome data collection is not as mysterious as once assumed.

Technical Assistance

If a project manager needs to hire additional staff to input data or manage patients or needs to pay for statistical or research design consultation, it is important to budget that into the costs of an outcome study. Paid consultants may be expensive, but they may also save a tremendous amount of time by shaping a good question to answer, designing the study, and designing the data collection processes. Statistical consultation may be necessary at the beginning of a project, to ensure that data are collected in a manner that is analyzable, and afterwards to conduct analyses. A statistician can look at whether the chosen variables will generate the answers of interest and thus save a project manager a lot of time in the developing stages.

One way to minimize the costs of performing data collection is to collaborate with local physical therapy programs, colleges, and universities. The expertise of the faculty (both physical therapy and non–physical therapy faculty) as well as access to graduate students who are looking for clinical or managerial research projects may be a cost-efficient solution for both parties.

Extending a Study

Assuming that the project manager has been successful in developing consensus for collecting data, the manager also needs to be prepared for the impact of a study's results. In Chapter 8, the rationale and possible outcomes for a study were identified. More than likely, the results will support one of the expected outcomes, and implementing change will seem like a natural next step.

Sometimes the results of data analyses do not support the expected outcomes, and they are not explained by the study's design or unique patient sample. In this situation, the project manager (and possibly others) must look to other sources of information to explain the results. This may mean reviewing procedures thoroughly, spending time observing practice patterns, or revisiting the literature. Any of these activities will require additional time.

Through this process, the investigating clinicians may see other ways to answer the original question. They may want to perform additional analyses of the data or collect additional data. These activities may lead to an extension of the original methods, collection of additional data, or revision of the data coding, resulting in reanalysis of recoded data.

> *There is great truth to the saying that "the more you learn, the more you realize how little you know."*

Even when the results are the ones expected or anticipated, the project manager must always be concerned about whether these results would be found consistently or whether the findings are coincidental. Replication or continued sampling of additional patient documentation is essential when the sample size is small in order to increase confidence in the results.

IMPLEMENTING CHANGES

Change Is Challenging

Most will agree that to collect and analyze patient data without acting on the less flattering findings would be a great waste of energy and expense; thus, change becomes part of the outcome measurement process. When areas that need improvement are identified from the results of a study, the next step is to create a plan for implementing changes. These changes may have an impact on documentation processes, intervention strategies, use of personnel, or how clinicians relate to patients. Any of these changes will require training so that everyone understands the nature of the problems and the solutions that will be attempted. The skills necessary to carry out the changes can be taught.

Staff reactions to change may range from enthusiastic support to overt denial and no desire to cooperate. Even under the best circumstances, those in management roles will need to anticipate the level of habit that staff have for a process that will be changed and the best ways to support everyone's efforts while making the changes. It will be important to convey to staff that changes made during one phase may be changed yet again as new information from additional outcome studies guides everyone toward providing the highest quality of service. This appreciation of on-going self-reflection is the basis of evidence-based improvement. Truly, there is no end to the measurement of clinical effectiveness!

Outcome Measurement Is an Ongoing Process

Performing an outcome study that looks only once at service effectiveness or cost does not allow the clinician to interpret these findings with much confidence. Multiple measures are needed for a clinician to understand if the results are due to seasonal changes, historical changes, or some unique way that data was collected.

To validate the findings of any investigation, whether it is basic science or clinical outcomes research, the scientific community requires that all studies must be reproducible. This means that the same facility should be able to produce similar results again or that others can produce similar results given similar conditions and using the same methods. If the results of a study are of concern, then it may be important to repeat the data collection on a second sample of patients. If the second set of results is different from the first set, then it will be important to identify whether the first sample had some unique biases or confounding conditions or whether both data sets represent very real levels of variability, such that both are valid reflections of practice. A third sampling may even be recommended.

As suggested above, outcome studies that produce less than pleasing results should spur changes in practice, but the goals for change should be measurable. It would be short-sighted to institute changes in practice without measuring the effectiveness of those changes through continued follow-up. Whether it is to validate prior results or to measure the effects of new changes, this serial approach to measurement and change becomes a management process of its own.

SECRETS TO SUCCESS

Keep It Simple

One of the greatest challenges faced at the start of any study is that of keeping it simple. A single patient or practice issue is inherently made complex by the number of variables that affect it. For example, if a clinician wanted to describe patients with arthritis who are typically treated in the clinic, the type of arthritis, the stage of progression, previous interventions, patient age, reimbursement source, referral source, gender, presenting symptoms, types of interventions, or measured changes in status could all be coded. These types of data support frequency analyses for each variable, and descriptions of clientele are needed according to levels of severity, amount of impairment change relative to reimbursement or types of intervention, or medical histories prior to seeking treatment. This is a lot of information. Thus, the single issue of describing a select group of patients in a practice will require codification of many variables.

Balance "Necessary" With "Interesting"

One of the struggles in designing an outcome study is sorting out the information that is *needed* from the information that is *interesting*. While this is difficult for the solo investigator, it is especially difficult when more than one person is involved in the study's design. Each person brings a slightly different perspective to the question of what should be studied. In the attempt to rally everyone's support, it is easy to consider answering several related questions; however, the downside of this strategy is that each additional question often requires documentation on many additional variables. If a clinician's primary role in a clinical setting is that of data collection, this may not be an issue.

Most clinical environments do not yet support full-time clinical researchers, and thus the data collection process will fall on the clinicians themselves. Documentation on 15 to 20 variables can add more time to a patient's visit. As clinician and client time are limited, there are three default options that may occur. Clinicians who are documenting patient status may need to decrease their patient loads; additional documentation may be squeezed into the current schedule, and rushing to complete it may result in inaccurate or incomplete documentation; surveys completed by patients may not be completed fully or correctly if patients perceive that their time is being wasted. Thus, keeping initial efforts simple may increase the ability to answer a question in a reasonable amount of time, may decrease the number of staff members who need to be trained in new documentation processes, and may decrease the overall documentation time for eligible patients.

Choose an Outcome Study With Confidence

The field of outcome measurement is wide open, even within the subset of retrospective studies. Most new investigations are primarily dedicated to accurately describing what exists (descriptive studies) before any specific variables are selected for change. Although much work has been done in measuring impairments, it reflects only one outcome of service delivery. There are also studies that evaluate functional outcomes from the rehabilitation perspective (e.g., Fetters & Kluzik, 1996) as well as from the patient's perspective. The latter includes studies on patient satisfaction and its relationship to clinical outcomes (e.g. Kane, Maciejewski, & Finch, 1997) and quality of life changes (e.g., Jette & Downing, 1996). Clinicians who venture into outcome measurements of their own practice patterns should rest assured that there are no wrong issues to study and there are no perspectives on issues that are needed more than others. Studies from all perspectives on all issues need to be addressed, so the clinician should address whatever is immediately important to daily practice.

SUMMARY

This chapter describes many of the managerial issues that need to be considered if changes in practice are implemented that affect people other than the investigating clinician. Issues of staff cooperation, training, and costs of conducting outcome measurements are reviewed. Even though there are many issues to be considered, clinicians should know that the processes of outcome measurement of any pertinent clinical issues that can clarify or improve their own service delivery are valuable and should be attempted. Clinicians will learn from the processes as well as the results!

References

Baker CM, Miller I, Sitterding M, & Hajewski CJ (1998). Acute stroke patients comparing outcomes with and without case management. Nursing Case Management 3(5):196–203.

Fetters L & Kluzik J (1996). The effects of neurodevelopmental treatment versus practice on the reaching of children with spastic cerebral palsy. Physical Therapy 76(4):346–358.

Focus on Therapeutic Outcomes, Inc., PO Box 11444, Knoxville, TN 37030 (fotoinc.com/frontis.htm).

Jette DU & Downing J (1996). The relationship of cardiovascular and psychological impairments to the health status of patients enrolled in cardiac rehabilitation programs. Physical Therapy 76(2):130–139.

Kane RL, Maciejewski M, & Finch M (1997). The relationship of patient satisfaction with care and clinical outcomes. Medical Care 35(7):714–730.

Kim S, et al. (2003). Effectiveness of clinical pathways for total knee and total hip arthroplasty: Literature review. Journal of Arthroplasty 18(1):69–74.

Koval KJ, et al. (2004). Clinical pathway for hip fractures in the elderly: the Hospital for Joint Diseases experience. Clinical Orthopaedics & Related Research 425:72–81.

Russek L, et al. (1997). Attitudes toward standardized data collection. Physical Therapy 77:714–729.

Thomas K (2003). Clinical pathway for hip and knee arthroplasty. Physiotherapy 89(10):603–609.

Uniform Data System for Medical Rehabilitation, a division of UB Foundation Activities, Inc. 270 Northpointe Parkway, Amherst NY (udsmr.org).

Wee AS, et al. (2000). The development of a stroke clinical pathway: An experience in a medium-sized community hospital. Journal of the Mississippi State Medical Association 41(7):648–653.

Mixing Outcome Measurement With Practice Management

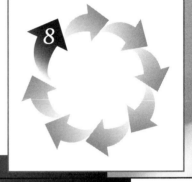

14

8

KEY TERMS

Quality assurance

Small qa

Large QA

Continuous Quality Improvement

Total Quality Management

Clinical pathways

Care paths

Protocols

Practice guidelines

Benchmarking

CHAPTER OUTCOMES

➤ Differentiate among the levels of quality assurance and management approaches.

➤ Relate the processes of outcome measurement to the processes of quality improvement.

➤ Describe the application of outcome measurement to development of clinical pathways.

➤ Relate the role of benchmarking to outcome measurement.

The focus of this book has been on the use of outcome measurement to improve the quality of one clinician's practice; that is, to develop an individual's skills as a reflective practitioner. Previous chapters introduced some of the ways that outcome data can influence daily practice routines, professional development, and documentation processes in a single setting. This chapter shifts the focus from the individual practitioner to a system of service delivery. It introduces quality assurance processes that ensure ongoing, cyclical review of practice expectations. The focus of data collection is expanded to include multiple outcomes, or collection of data from multiple clinicians. It is then used for ongoing internal review, for development of clinical pathways or guidelines, and for benchmarking against known standards of excellence.

QUALITY ASSURANCE

Quality assurance is a process used to monitor whether predetermined standards of service delivery are met in daily practice. The standards may reflect expectations for documentation or procedural routines. Typical documentation standards include recording such items as the date of an evaluation, a patient's referral source, and the signature and license number of the therapist. Examples of documented procedural routines include annual safety electrical inspections of machines, application of universal precautions, and training staff in Health Insurance Portability and Accountability Act regulations.

For most documentation formats, a checklist of the expected practice standards is developed, and medical records are reviewed against that checklist. Rates of missing or incorrectly recorded items are calculated to determine if adequate levels of compliance have been met.

Quality assurance processes have traditionally emphasized the correction of errors or the identification of poor performers. They do not typically address the processes that underlie the errors (Coleman & Endsley, 1999; McKinley, et al., 1998). Checklists for documentation standards are easily constructed from practice standards published by professional or accrediting organizations or by government agencies. Record reviews often happen in locations separate from practice locations, such as in records departments or conference rooms. Thus, knowledge of the processes contributing to frequent errors is not likely to be reviewed.

The parties that set standards for practice vary. They include individuals and/or administrators within a practice setting, external organizations such as accrediting bodies, and government regulatory agencies. Settings such as a hospital department may have practice standards defined by several of these parties.

Chart reviews may be conducted by a clinician from within the clinical setting, or they may be performed by an external reviewer. When reviewers come from within the organization, they may be able to detect errors as well as recommend solutions to prevent future errors. When reviewers come from outside, they may not know enough about how a department functions to make recommendations that will work.

Small qa Versus Large QA

De Geyndt (1970) separates quality assurance (QA) processes into two distinct levels. **Small qa** focuses primarily on the structure of the activity; it is initiated after a problem is identified to determine minimum levels of compliance or competence. An example is when a group of billings is denied because a particular item of information has not been recorded on a form. Once the frequency of the problem is identified, a procedure for correction can be instituted, and subsequent documentation reviews can measure whether compliance is improving.

Large QA has a broader focus. This process addresses the presence or absence of compliance with standards as well as the *reasons* for variation. When a problem is identified, a cause for the problem is sought in addition to setting an expected outcome. Consumers may be consulted or interviewed, and utilization routines may be observed or reviewed. In the end, solutions are suggested that will promote higher levels of effectiveness and efficiency related to the problem. Additionally, there is commitment to ongoing evaluation regarding the initial problem (Fig. 14.1)

Continuous Quality Improvement

Continuous Quality Improvement (CQI) is the ongoing process of measuring the quality of services provided and making the services more effective (Coleman & Endsley, 1999; McIntosh, May, & Stymiest, 1994.) It builds on de Geyndt's (1970) concept of large QA as it emphasizes understanding and improvement of the foundational work processes or routines (McKinley, et al., 1998).

Principles of CQI address customer satisfaction, procedures for continuous improvement, involvement of the entire organization such that everyone perceives a sense of ownership, and use of data and provider knowledge to improve decision-making (McKinley, et al., 1998; Coleman & Endsley, 1999). Unlike small qa processes, in which the standards are often determined by outside agencies to protect the public, the perspective of CQI is first and foremost on seeking to improve customer satisfaction. The CQI process has traditionally been conducted at the managerial level.

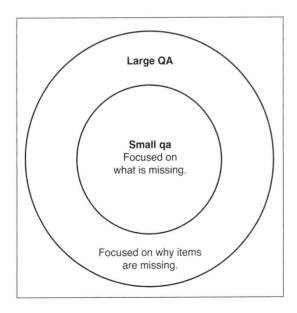

Figure 14.1 Small qa versus large QA.

For example, customer satisfaction is improved by enabling a patient to achieve the maximum benefit in the least amount of time, for the least amount of money, and in the most comfortable manner. Patient satisfaction surveys often address multiple aspects of service delivery and can provide the patient's perspective on the quality and outcomes of services. The challenge, as described in Chapter 2, Common Outcomes in Rehabilitation, is to identify the one or two variables that affect patient satisfaction that, with improvement, will improve overall care. As there are many aspects that contribute to patient satisfaction, CQI processes are helpful because they establish an ongoing, systematic look at how service is delivered (Fig. 14.2).

Total Quality Management

Total Quality Management (TQM) is a participatory and systematic approach to planning and implementing continuous organizational improvement focused on customer satisfaction (Kaluzny, McLaughlin, & Simpson, 1992). In contrast to CQI, which is typically initiated at the managerial level, TQM processes can begin with any service provider who recognizes opportunities for improvement. This includes employees and volunteers, whether they are directly interacting with the patient (such as clinicians) or indirectly supporting patient care (such as medical records or housekeeping staff). Everyone with a role in the delivery of services is included in an ongoing process of quality improvement (Fig. 14.3).

FIVE AREAS TO MEASURE

CQI and TQM essentially serve the same purpose: to improve the services that contribute to customer or patient satisfaction. The essential difference relates to who has responsibility for initiating the evaluation of issues or identifying suggestions for improvement. In either approach, there are five areas of service delivery that can be measured (de Geyndt, 1970).

Structure refers to the qualifications and credentials of the staff and the physical structures in which services are delivered. In the case of rehabilitation staff, qualifications might include current licensure, CPR certification, and specialist certification. The physical structures include the adequacy and appropriateness of the clinic space. A facility that serves only adults with sport-related injuries will naturally be different than what is appropriate for infants and young children, and those environments will be different from a clinic that serves all ages.

Process refers to what actually happens during the course of service delivery. Observations are made to describe what the clinician does, what the

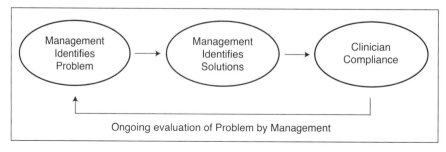

Figure 14.2 CQI processes are traditionally managerial responsibilities.

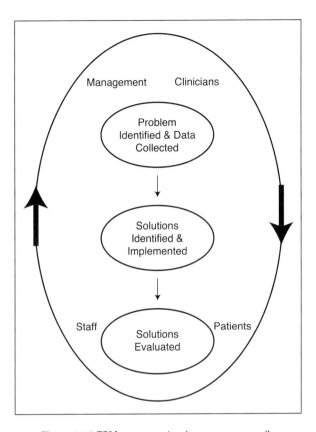

Figure 14.3 TQM processes involve everyone equally.

patient does, and what supportive service people provide. Patterns of movement in and out of the clinical areas, patient scheduling, patient interviews, and the frequency and reasons for equipment use are examples of processes that can be studied.

Outcome measurement focuses primarily on patient results. Patient results include such outcomes as changes in impairments, function and participation, satisfaction with services, the environment and patient perceptions of improvement, long-term outcomes, and need for additional episodes of care for the same problem.

Content evaluation focuses on the appropriateness of care. Evaluators look at issues such as whether patient problems are linked to service utilization; patterns of care that are incorrect or unnecessary; or, conversely, patterns of care that describe best practice.

Impact measurement focuses on a much broader outcome: the impact of care on society. In this case, the overall effectiveness of service delivery is viewed in terms of who is served, who is not served, and whether services enhance the quality of life for recipients. Such measures might include rates of return to work, the cost benefits of providing preventative services to a corporation, or the communities of people who have access to services.

STEPS OF CQI/TQM

CQI/TQM processes follow the same steps as those of an outcome study for a single practitioner. The scale is larger, and there may be more variables to measure, but the basic steps follow the cyclical process that individual outcome studies follow: a problem is identified and quantified through a measurement process, an intervention is imposed to improve the initial baseline, and remeasurement occurs.

Step 1: Identify Problems

The Model of Rehabilitation Service Delivery presented in Chapter 6 serves as a useful organizer for identifying quality assurance issues. CQI/TQM processes can evaluate problems related to any part of the service delivery process. *Inputs*, such as the geographic area served, the number of physicians referring to the service, or the preparation of clinicians that serve the patients, can be evaluated. Examples of measurable *processes* include scheduling efficiency, documentation and medical record management, and utilization of interventions. Examples of *outcomes* include patients' perceptions about whether their expectations have been met, whether they feel their health status has improved as a result of services received, or whether they are satisfied with their experiences at a facility. All these examples should sound familiar as they are studies that can be conducted on a single clinician's caseload as a reflective practitioner. The difference between studying an issue as a reflective practitioner versus a CQI/TQM process is that the former involves the records of just one practitioner. CQI/TQM involves the records of many service providers and input from those who receive the services. Whether an issue is evaluated as an individual outcome study or as part of CQI/TQM, the two processes are cyclical activities of evaluation, modification of process, and reevaluation of outcomes.

Step 2: Select a Priority for Improvement and Define Variables

After areas for improvement are identified, a priority goal is targeted for improvement. The variables describing the goal are identified and operationally defined. This process of operationally defining the variables of interest is the same as for individual outcome studies. The literature should be consulted for existing definitions, and a coding handbook should be developed. Development of the coding handbook is more extensive as there will be more variables to track and more people who must understand and agree with the operational definitions. In CQI/TQM processes, where many are involved in the delivery of services, expected behaviors or routines should be clearly delineated so that everyone knows what to evaluate and how to change the process.

Step 3: Collect Data

Once the variables or behaviors have been defined, baseline data are collected to quantify the current level of performance. Data collection can take place through a variety of mechanisms. CQI/TQM processes are interested in the extent of the problem *and* the cause of the problem. Therefore, it is important to collect quantitative data on the frequency of the problem as well as qualitative data on the causes of problems. Qualitative data may be derived from interviews, surveys, or focus groups and should include both the service providers and patients involved in the process. The goal of this step is to gain input from everyone who may have insight into the problem, its causes, and possible solutions. This type of data collection is slightly different from the purely objective or quantitative data collection that individual retrospective outcome studies might focus on. In CQI/TQM studies, understanding why a problem exists, what processes contribute to the problem, and what processes enhance the desired goal all need to be described.

Step 4: Analyze Causes of Key Problems

Once data have been collected on the key issue, the causes of the problems are identified. Triangulation is the process of comparing data from multiple sources to see where common explanations or descriptions arise as well as where there are conflicting explanations. Inconsistencies among the data sources are red flags that different perceptions exist or that there are mismatches between expected practice and actual practice.

For example, a CQI/TQM team interested in increasing the frequency of documentation on functional goals could collect data from medical *charts reviews*, from *interviews* with therapists, and from *observations* of practice. The patient records may reflect inconsistent documentation about changes in functional skills, whereas the interviews with therapists might indicate a strong commitment to functionally oriented goals. The patient records might provide *objective data* on the frequency of documentation but will not shed light on why the documentation is inconsistent. *Interviews* with clinicians might indicate a variety of reasons, such as a lack of time to document function, lack of space on the forms, inability to quantify individual goals of patients, or a lack of knowledge about available measurement tools. *Observations* might suggest that the clinicians have inadequate workspace to complete documentation or that forms are not conveniently located. Based on these three forms of data collection (chart review, interview, and observation), trends in behaviors, environmental conditions, and frequency of the targeted behavior are identified to form the basis for solutions.

Step 5: Develop Solutions and Set Goals

Potential solutions may be identified at any time: during problem identification, during data collection, and after data collection. Everyone's observations can give rise to ideas and strategies for correction. From these ideas and other brainstorming sessions with the team, one or several viable solutions are derived that may be put into action.

Measurable goals are set for the expected performance. Sometimes, setting goals is as simple as exceeding a baseline; in other cases, the goal is a targeted level of performance. Determining what an acceptable target is may need to be the result of a consensus process. In this way, everyone contributes to determining a reasonable level of improvement based on the viable solutions. Having a target or a specific measurement to achieve or exceed is critical for focusing everyone's efforts.

Step 6: Implement and Monitor

The final step is to implement a solution or set of solutions and measure the affect on the expected outcomes. It is important to assign someone to oversee the implementation process. This person may be directly involved in the use of the solution or removed from the process. Outcome monitoring should follow timelines to ensure periodic evaluation of a solution's effectiveness.

It is important and motivating to provide feedback about the success of the solution(s). Feedback to service providers at regular intervals helps to keep everyone aware of the goal and their progress toward it. It helps to identify whether there are unexpected problems implementing the plan and provides everyone with opportunities to alter the strategy midstream.

CQI/TQM processes are ongoing, so repeated measurement provides scheduled feedback about the consistency of the improved performance over a long period. As outcomes improve, understanding of the issues improves, and new solutions can be implemented to achieve even higher targets for the same goals. Thus, the cyclical process of continual improvement becomes a routine part of clinical practice.

The ultimate outcome of CQI/TQM is the identification of those steps or methods of service delivery that consistently yield the best results for that outcome. In other words, the ultimate outcome of continuous improvement is the definition of best practice in that facility. When best practice is defined around the management of patients, it is the basis for developing effective clinical pathways within that clinical setting.

CLINICAL PATHWAYS, CARE PATHS, AND PROTOCOLS

Clinical pathways, sometimes called critical pathways, outline the agreed-upon steps for the diagnosis and management of a condition or procedure for individual patients. They specify the interdisciplinary services to be delivered, the timing of the services, and the responsible parties for those services (Harkleroad, et al., 2000; Weiland, 1997). They are predominantly management tools based on clinical information gathered from patient records, outcome studies, or other guidelines or parameters. They may be developed within an institution by a committee or adapted from commercially available publications and Web site postings.

Clinical pathways are specific to the institution using them because they are tailored to the unique characteristics of the service delivery environment and culture (American Academy of Physical Medicine and Rehabilitation, 2000). Even when they are adopted from published guidelines, the unique aspects of service delivery patterns in a particular setting need to be incorporated into the path in order for it to work. For example, a clinical pathway might have a step that refers the patient to a medical social worker. That might work in institution A, but if that responsibility is handled by a nurse case manager in institution B, the pathway will need to be adapted. Figure 14.4 is an example of a portion of a clinical pathway for patients with hip fracture.

Care paths are the documentation mechanisms that indicate if the clinical pathway has been followed. They may include timelines, plans, management, and evaluation processes. They are forms with areas designated for documentation about each step of a critical pathway. The individual assigned to each step notes that the activity has been implemented or, if delayed, the reasons for that.

Clinical pathways are used to reduce variability and cost, increase efficiency, and monitor and improve patient care (Bertholf, 1998; Harkleroad, et al., 2000; Weiland, 1997). They are linked to the CQI/TQM process because

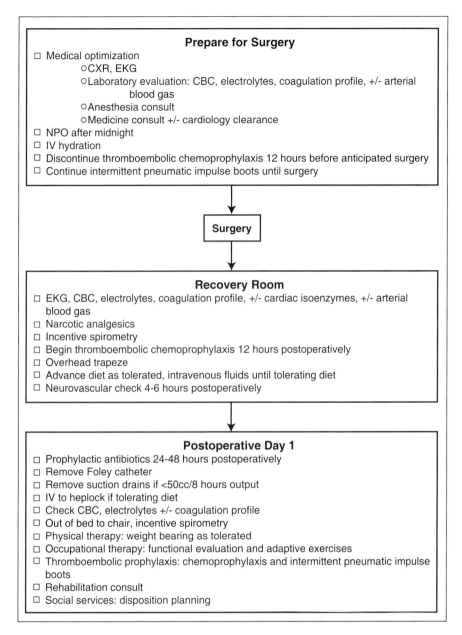

Figure 14.4 Example of a portion of a clinical pathway for hip fracture. (From Koval KJ, et al [2004]. Clinical pathway for hip fractures in the elderly. Clinical Orthopaedics and Related Research 425:72-81.)

CQI/TQM requires the description of routine activities in order to improve the activities. Once a procedural problem is defined, measured, altered, and measured again, it is reasonable to convert the more effective process into a pathway that all clinicians can follow.

Clinical pathways are different from **patient care protocols**. A clinical pathway is an overview or general plan of actions or tasks for the overall management of a particular patient group. It reflects the activities of *multiple disciplines* or service providers and does not specify the details of the task to be performed. Protocols typically relate to the progression of a specific intervention for a particular diagnostic group; they are initiated by a service provider within a *specific discipline*. For example, a patient receiving a total hip replacement will receive care from many different health-care providers. A clinical pathway would identify the actions for which each discipline is responsible and when those actions would generally occur within that specific institution. For example, physical therapy would be identified to perform a postoperative evaluation on day 1 or continue therapy for days 2 to 7. In contrast, a protocol for total hip rehabilitation would be a discipline-specific plan of care for the physical therapist to follow. It would specify the precautions and progression of exercises, weight-bearing status, and educational topics that should be addressed on each day of rehabilitation.

Development and use of a clinical pathway does not absolve clinicians from using sound clinical judgment (Sheehan, 2002). Clinical pathways are just guidelines for care that have been tailored to a specific institution. The clinician will need to determine if each patient's status is consistent with progressing to the next step of a clinical pathway or whether there are contraindications to continuing.

Examples of the Effectiveness of Clinical Pathways

Three studies are presented to illustrate the effectiveness of using clinical pathways for patient care. All three have rehabilitation-related outcomes for patient populations that are commonly managed by physical therapists.

Healy, et al. (1998) studied the effect of implementing a clinical pathway and hip implantation protocol for total hip arthroplasty on patient satisfaction, surgical outcomes, and complication rates. Patient outcomes were measured from 89 procedures performed before implementation of the clinical pathway and 117 procedures after implementation. There were no differences between the groups on any patient related outcomes; however, use of the clinical pathway and hip protocol reduced the length and cost of the hospital stay.

Shaldach (1997) compared the effects of using a clinical pathway for patients with lower extremity amputations. Group 1 had no clinical pathway, group 2 had a clinical pathway with a consult to rehabilitation services, and group 3 used a rehabilitation-focused pathway. The study demonstrated that the referral to rehabilitation reduced hospital stays by approximately 3 days, that more patients from group 3 went home than for groups 1 and 2, and that the use of a rehabilitation-focused clinical pathway was more cost-effective than a general pathway with a referral for rehabilitation services.

Mehta, et al. (2000) compared patient management outcomes before and after implementation of a clinical pathway for 497 patients diagnosed with myocardial infarction. The pathway was designed to increase adherence to service delivery standards by multiple health-care professionals. Adherence to many medical management practices was increased substantially, including an increase in referrals for outpatient rehabilitation. Patient education provided as part of the services in the pathway was correlated positively with greater adherence to medication use and participation in outpatient rehabilitation.

In summary, the implementation of clinical pathways can be effective in reducing variation and replication of services, reducing length of stay and overall cost of management, and for increasing interdisciplinary management of patient care.

Developing a Clinical Pathway

There are several circumstances for which the development of clinical pathways would be useful for an individual physical therapy department or clinic. If a clinic has a **high patient volume** for a specific diagnosis or type of patient, a clinical pathway may help to streamline the management of those patients. This is particularly true if multiple therapists are involved in the management of individual patients, or if there are wide variations in the management of similar patients.

When a **high level of risk** for a negative outcome exists, a clinical pathway may ensure that selective precautionary activities are routinely implemented. These activities might include documentation of specific types of information, use of particular types of educational procedures, or provision of protective equipment and instructions for their use.

When the **cost of care** for a type of patient is high, a clinical pathway may help to contain the overall management costs by identifying when certain procedures should occur and by whom. Redundant steps or replication of services is consequently diminished, which contributes to cost containment.

Sheehan (2002) recommends that all clinical pathways should be well documented. They should have a title, list the developers, reference all the literature and sources reviewed to develop the plan, identify all those who reviewed the pathway, verify that the pathway does not conflict with policies, and describe all meetings, procedures, documentation responsibilities, and in-services that are involved. By documenting all the steps of development and all procedures for implementation, the clinic is better prepared to use the pathway responsibly.

Practice Guidelines

Practice guidelines are recommendations for patient management that are not unique to any institution. They may be developed by an institution, but generally they are developed by organizations or study groups. Practice guidelines are established to improve patient outcomes, reduce wrongful management of patient conditions, control costs, and inform patients and clinicians about appropriate choices for medical management (Scalzitti, 2001; Woolf, 1992). Woolf (1992) describes four levels of guidelines.

- **Informal consensus development** is based on expert opinion without specific methods used to evaluate related literature.
- **Formal consensus development** is based on a structured opportunity to develop guidelines. Different organizations, such as the National Institutes of Health Consensus Development Program (consensus.nih.gov) and the Rand Corporation (rand.org), have created structured opportunities for expert panels to meet in order to develop guidelines on the management of selected medical issues. While the time and format of the documents are structured to ensure consistency from one conference meeting to the next, integration of literature to support the guideline development is variable.
- **Evidence-based guidelines** integrate the available literature and expert clinical opinion. The methods and structure of the literature review process as well as the amount of expert opinion vary, depending on the supporting organization.

- **Explicit guidelines** specify the benefits, harms, financial costs, and the probability of selected outcomes of procedures and interventions. They are based on literature and expert opinion, and the relative contribution of each source is acknowledged.

Access to clinical guidelines is growing quickly due to the Internet. The Agency for Healthcare Research and Quality (AHRQ) (ahrq.gov) is a government agency that focuses on health-care services research. Its website provides access to reports on current and past research. The AHRQ developed a series of 19 clinical guidelines published between 1992 and 1996. These guidelines are available online through the AHRQ website (ahrq.gov/clinic/cpgonline). Although some of these may be outdated, they provide a strong foundation for understanding the structure and organization of an extensive guideline. Moreover, many of the guidelines focus on patients or conditions managed by physical therapists. For example, there are guidelines on management of acute low back pain, cardiac rehabilitation, pressure ulcer prevention and treatment, and management of pain or depression.

The National Guideline Clearinghouse (NGC) (guidelines.gov), operated by the US Department of Health and Human Services, is a database of evidence-based clinical guidelines. Jointly supported by AHRQ, the American Medical Association, and the American Association of Health Plans, NGC provides access to a large collection of guidelines developed by a variety of sources. Visitors to this website can search the database with simple terms, compare two or more guidelines in a side-by-side layout, and print the results. Visitors are warned that the NGC makes no attempt to review the quality of the posted guidelines as long as all requirements for submission have been met.

International efforts to establish and disseminate guidelines are growing and are readily accessible through the Internet. The Guidelines International Network (g-i-n.net) has 61 organizations from 33 countries contributing to its efforts to identify, develop, and disseminate medical guidelines. The Canadian Medical Association (CMA) supports the CMA INFOBASE (mdm.ca/cpgsnew/cpgs/index.asp), a searchable resource of clinical practice guidelines. Many CMA guidelines are available in two versions, one for health-care professionals and one as a patient guide. The Centre for Evidence Based Physiotherapy (cebp.nl) in the Netherlands maintains a list of guidelines and links to other sources specific to physical therapy.

There are many special interest groups that publish guidelines or post them on their websites. The National Heart, Lung, and Blood Institute (nhlbi.nih.gov/guidelines) posts guidelines on asthma management. The Workers Compensation Board of British Columbia Canada has published literature-based, postoperative rehabilitation guidelines on its website (worksafebc.com). Topics include anterior cruciate ligament reconstruction, carpal tunnel release, and simple and complex meniscectomies. The October 2001 edition of *Physical Therapy* was devoted to the presentation of evidence-based guidelines developed by the Philadelphia Panel on management of patients with low back, knee, neck, and shoulder pain. Clinicians and researchers systematically reviewed the available literature to determine the presence and strength of evidence for common interventions. Expert Clinical Benchmarks (expertclinicalbenchmarks.com) is a for-profit company that uses expert opinion, literature review, and proprietary data to develop guidelines that are made available to the public.

In the absence of an established guideline, Megens and Harris (1999) applied evidence-based practice principles to develop guidelines for the management of lymphedema following breast cancer. This article demonstrates how literature is collected, critically appraised, and then summarized to suggest guidelines for clinical decision-making.

BENCHMARKING

Benchmarking Definitions

Benchmarking is the process of comparing one's own procedures and outcomes with those of a known or best available *gold standard* in order to improve consumer or client service outcomes. The Benchmarking Network (2000) defines it as "a performance measurement tool used in conjunction with improvement initiatives to measure comparative operating performance and identify Best Practices." A slightly different definition of benchmarking is "the continuous process of measuring products, services and practices against the toughest competitors and those companies recog nized as industry leaders" (David T. Kerns, former CEO, Xerox Corp., from Russell, 1998).

In both definitions, the intention is to compare current performance against the performance of a person or company that has a known record of excellence. That record of excellence sets a gold standard for its competition by defining best practice at that time. The key to being recognized as a gold standard is the ability to *consistently* demonstrate a high level of performance that results in high consumer satisfaction.

Levels of Benchmarking

There are different levels at which benchmarking occurs. At the **staff level**, clinicians can identify best practice outcomes from within an organization and strive to have all clinicians at that level. This often occurs informally when new graduates are hired into a practice setting where more experienced therapists are working. Common benchmarks include the numbers of patients treated per day or the timely completion of paperwork; however, these standards are important to the management and not so important to the consumer.

Benchmarking can be applied at the staff level to patient care. Data are emerging on the expected benchmarks for recovery of patients with select diagnoses. Stineman, et al. (1998) described median performance levels for 18 functional tasks recorded on the Functional Independence Measure for 9 levels of disability in 26,339 patients with strokes. This type of data allows individual therapists and rehabilitation departments to compare their own outcomes against a larger cohort and provides evidence for predicting outcomes more accurately.

Benchmarking at the staff level requires defining an aspect of service delivery, identifying who best delivers that aspect of practice and *how* they do it, and then training staff to emulate those best practices. That benchmark may be a person who already works within the department or someone external to the department who has a record of excellent outcomes. Regardless of who is chosen as the benchmark, the expected changes in practice are measurable, and success is marked by positive changes in patient-related outcomes.

Benchmarking also occurs **interdepartmentally** within a large organization. In this case, rather than comparing individual staff members with other staff members, departments are compared with other departments in the organization. A common organizational benchmark is consumer or patient satisfaction rating. In a hospital setting, satisfaction may be rated by the patient for every professional service received. At selected times, patient satisfaction ratings are calculated, and departments are compared with one another by the organization's administration. In this situation, the gold standard may be a set criterion (such as a 95% satisfaction ratings for all departments), may be relative to whichever department is highest at the time of reporting, or may be relative to the past performance of the same department. At this level, benchmarking in an internal process within the organization, with target performance levels set by the organization.

Benchmarking more traditionally occurs between **agreeing parties from different organizations**. In this case, a person or organization is identified as the gold standard with a consistently excellent outcome that many want to emulate. The benchmark person or organization is approached; the procedures of the benchmark person/practice are described and compared with those of the clinic. Differences are identified, and decisions are made about whether the benchmark practices can be implemented and to what extent. It is possible to identify many differences but only implement a few procedural changes.

The real challenge is to identify the benchmark! The person or clinic must have objective evidence to support the perceptions of being a gold standard for the desired outcome. That evidence should indicate that there is a *history* of excellence rather than a recent success as there are many variables that can affect patient care statistics. However, whereas a business may be reluctant to share the secrets of its success with a local competitor, it may be willing to share its methods with a practice with which it is not in direct competition.

Benchmarking can be performed against a **known set of standards**. LaClair, et al. (2001) compared the process of care provided to stroke patients at 11 Veterans Administration hospitals with that of the Agency for Health Care Policy and Research Post-Stroke Rehabilitation Clinical Practice Guidelines. LaClair, et al. developed a measurement system that reflected guideline compliance and sampled 100 patient records. The results described the areas of greatest and least compliance, thus establishing baselines for service review. In this type of benchmarking process, it is assumed that the chosen guidelines represent current best practice. The primary limitation of this type of benchmarking is that the strategies for achieving best practice are not available for study. Guidelines represent a composite of many sources and are meant to be general recommendations, so the strategies for matching the guideline recommendations will need to be developed within the organization rather than by emulating another setting.

Benchmarking Steps

The steps for benchmarking build on the processes of outcome measurement and continuous quality improvement. Benchmarking at the individual level will be less complex than benchmarking within an organization, and that is less complex than benchmarking against a different organization. At each level, more people and more communication are involved, but there are many rewards from studying and implementing strategies that result in best practice patterns. The following is a brief description of the benchmarking process.

Step 1: Assemble a team to develop a project plan. The team will need to have a project leader to organize the process. While familiarity with the benchmarking process is helpful, it is more important that the leader be experienced in group processes and facilitation. These skills are essential for ensuring cooperation from the many people involved in the process. Like all team efforts, the project team will function more smoothly if it consists of a small group of congenial people who are focused on a similar goal. Therefore, it helps to have a mission statement that clearly articulates the goals of the team. The team should represent a variety of needs, practices, and points of view relative to the process being studied. This will improve the team's ability to create a true and full description of its own practices before comparing itself with others. A benchmarking team is more successful when it defines success by improvements in the organization or department, rather than looking for successful performance of individual team members. To facilitate this team approach, it may be helpful to have the project team receive training on the purpose of the benchmarking process and strategies for implementing a study.

The project plan should grow out of a perceived need for improvement based on the data from departmental or institutional outcomes studies. The data should reflect a history of measurements taken over time rather than a single measurement. If that history of data is not available, then the team is probably not ready to begin benchmarking. If that history of data is available, it should reflect periods of change when procedures were implemented to improve the outcomes of interest. The history of what has been tried, what has worked, and what has not worked will help the team select the most appropriate areas to target for change and the most appropriate clinician or business to use as a benchmark.

Step 2: Describe the department's own processes for achieving its current level of outcomes. It is important to have a very clear understanding of current processes. If changes are recommended, it is necessary to know what steps in a process need to be altered.

Step 3: Identify a potential benchmark partner. This partner should have an established history of continued excellence in the process that the team is hoping to study and be agreeable to being a benchmark partner.

As a benchmark partner, there are several levels of interaction in which a clinician or business might be asked to engage. These levels include participating in meetings to describe strategies and data, opening their business to outside observers, and/or providing consultation, observation, and training in the team's setting. All these levels are predetermined as part of the project plan and benchmarking agreements.

Step 4: Develop an accurate description of the benchmark partner's processes. These descriptions are the basis from which to make comparisons. Once data have been collected on the benchmark partner's practices, the project team tries to determine where performance gaps exist between its own setting and that of the benchmark partner.

Step 5: Project goals are set. These are based on the most important performance gaps, and plans are developed to implement changes. Even though many differences between the two practices are identified, not all of them will need to be addressed. The goals should be measurable.

Step 6: The changes are monitored. The processes are evaluated at regular intervals, with repeated measures of the target outcome to determine if the processes are being executed and if the outcome is improving as anticipated.

Examples From the Literature

Novalis, Messenger, and Morris (1999) examined the occupational therapy benchmarks across eight multidisciplinary critical pathways for management of patients with total hip replacements. Frequency analysis of 14 roles of occupational therapists in the critical pathways demonstrated that training in activities of daily living was identified in all the pathways, but there was high variability in the remaining 13 roles. This study also identified that occupational therapy was included in total hip critical pathways with the same frequency as nursing and physical therapy. This type of study is useful for identifying the roles of a profession and is the first step toward clarifying practice patterns.

Simpson (2002) compared patients with hip fracture who participated in an early discharge/transitional care critical pathway with those receiving standard care. The results indicated that patients were generally satisfied with the overall care and clinical outcomes achieved with the critical pathway. Additionally, the use of community care services following early hospital discharge resulted in significant cost of care savings per patient as compared with those in the standard care group.

APPLICATIONS TO PRACTICE

The use of outcome data has been described as it relates to the processes of continuous quality improvement, development of clinical pathways, protocols and guidelines, and benchmarking. These processes are all related to the identification of best practice patterns. There are other reasons for conducting outcome studies of service delivery, regardless of whether it is at the individual, intraorganizational, or interorganizational level.

Through the use of outcome measurement and management processes, the strengths and development needs of the clinical staff become clarified. If selected interventions are studied or documentation processes are instituted, then management can focus *staff training* on those specific areas. For example, in a review of documentation processes, a practice may decide to implement the use of selected standardized measurement tools. Among the clinical staff, some may be more or less familiar with the use of the selected tools. By arranging for staff training on the use and scoring of the tools, management will increase compliance with the use of the tools as well as improve intra- and interrater reliability of the scoring.

Outcome data can be used to *market* the quality and efficiency of clinical services to the general public, to referral sources, and to third party payers. Use of outcome data on performance measures improves the accountability that patients are increasingly seeking. Many people receive their health and medical information from the media, so performance data that are presented on the Internet, in newspapers, or in radio or television interviews add credibility to the presentation (Scroggins, Thornton, & Neumann, 1999). One such example is Carepathways.com, which publishes nursing home inspection reports for each state.

There is growing use of institutional report cards, where the performance grades are updated on a regular schedule and published for distribution. Some clinics include these as pamphlets for patients to take home on their first visit. As consumers increasingly rely on the Internet, online rating services and referral sites are proliferating. Patients naturally choose to use those facilities with better patient satisfaction ratings and/or performance outcomes.

The physical therapy profession is constantly evolving in response to changes in health policy, economic forces, and advances in medical management. Outcome studies enable clinicians to replace the best practice patterns of the past with more efficient, even better practice patterns. As new developments in other patient management arenas emerge, such as in pharmacology, surgery, technology, and physiology, practice patterns will need to adjust and be retested for efficacy. Thus the cycle of improvement continues.

SUMMARY

This chapter provides an overview of outcome measurement processes as they relate to larger systematic studies of service delivery. Outcome study processes are related to those of quality assurance, CQI, TQM, and development of clinical pathways, protocols, and guidelines and their use for benchmarking against a known gold standard. The effort and commitment necessary for these processes yield the benefits of improving local practice, establishing best practice patterns, improving accountability to patients, providing marketing strategies for businesses, and moving the profession forward through publication of effective outcome management studies.

References

American Academy of Physical Medicine & Rehabilitation (2000). Practice Guidelines Committee develops definitions of terms. aapmr.org/memphys/pracguid/terms.htm.

Bertholf L (1998). Clinical pathways from conception to outcome. Top Health Information Management 19(2):30–34.

Coleman MT & Endsley S (1999). Quality improvement: First steps. Family Practice Management 3:23–26.

de Geyndt W (1970). Five approaches for assessing the quality of care. Hospital Administration 159:21–42.

Harkleroad A, Schirf D, Volpe J, & Holm MB (2000). Critical pathway development: An integrative literature review. American Journal of Occupational Therapy 54:148–154.

Healy WE, et al. (1998). Impact of a clinical pathway and implant standardization on total hip arthroplasty: A clinical and economic study of short-term patient outcome. Journal of Arthroplasty 13(3): 266–276.

Kaluzny AD, McLaughlin CP, & Simpson K (1992). Applying total quality management concepts to public health organizations. Public Health Reports 107(3):257–264.

Koval KJ, et al. (2004). Clinical pathway for hip fractures in the elderly. Clinical Orthopaedics and Related Research. 425:72–81.

LaClair BJ, et al. (2001). A method for measuring compliance with AHCPR guidelines. American Journal of Physical Medicine and Rehabilitation 80(3):235–242.

McIntosh G, May MC, & Stymiest PJ (1994). Implementing CQI: Measuring levels of service quality at physiotherapy clinics. Physiotherapy Canada. 46(3):178–189.

McKinley CO, et al. (1998). Performance improvement: The organization's quest. Journal of Rehabilitation Outcomes Measurement 2(1):27–35.

Megens A & Harris SR (1998). Physical therapist management of lymphedema following treatment for breast cancer: A critical literature review of its effectiveness. Physical Therapy 78:1302–1311.

Mehta RH, et al. (2000). Quality improvement initiative and its impact on the management of patients with acute myocardial infarction. Archives of Internal Medicine 160(20):3057–3062.

Novalis SD, Messenger MF, & Morris L (1999). Occupational therapy benchmarks within orthopedic (hip) critical pathways. American Journal of Occupational Therapy 54:155–158.

Russell P (1998). Looking beyond yourself: Benchmarking tools and techniques. Mayo Press, Mayo Medical Center, Rochester, MN.

Scalzitti DA (2001). Evidence-based guidelines: Application to clinical practice. Physical Therapy 81:1622–1628.

Schaldach DE (1997). Measuring quality and cost of care: Evaluation of an amputation clinical pathway. Journal of Vascular Nursing 15(1):13–20.

Scroggins N, Thornton S, & Neumann T (1999). Role of outcomes management in marketing to managed care companies: Why use outcomes data? Outcomes Management for Nursing Practice 3(1):7–11.

Sheehan JP (2002). A liability checklist for clinical pathways. Nursing Management 33(2):23–25.

Simpson P (2002). Clinical outcomes in transition program for older adults with hip fracture. Outcomes Management. 6(2):86–89.

Stineman MG, Fiedler RC, Granger CV, & Maislin G (1998). Functional task benchmarks for stroke rehabilitation. 79(5):497–504.

The Benchmarking Network (2000). well.com/user/benchmar/Files/General.html

Weiland DE (1997). Why use clinical pathways rather than practice guidelines? American Journal of Surgery 174(6):592–595.

Woolf SH (1992). Practice guidelines, a new reality in medicine: II. Methods of developing guidelines. Archives of Internal Medicine 152:946–952.

Conduct a Pilot Study of Documentation Patterns

This section will guide clinicians through a pilot study of their own documentation patterns.

This is a reasonable starting point for the clinician who would like to begin tracking outcomes in a practice setting. A study of documentation patterns will reveal whether patient characteristics or measures are recorded consistently. Inconsistent documentation will need to be addressed to establish a source of usable data before other clinical outcomes can be studied.

The steps of this study follow the explanations provided in Part 2, Chapters 7–12:

1. Identify an interest, and form the question (Chapter 7)
2. Conduct a search of the literature (Chapter 8)
3. Identify a rationale for conducting the study and potential action plans (Chapter 8)
4. Define relevant variable codes (Chapter 9)
5. Create a data set (Chapter 10)
6. Analyze the data (Chapter 11)
7. Interpret results, and create a report (Chapter 12)

You will be recording the disablement category of each goal and the measurability of each goal for the purpose of personal self-improvement in documentation practices. Other characteristics of documentation can be measured as well, but for a first study, it may be useful to limit data harvesting to the initial evaluation. For clinicians with more experience, consider whether a final measurement needs to be recorded for each goal set.

The study is limited to those records that were personally completed by the clinician conducting the study to accommodate HIPAA regulations. Be aware that for review of any records other than your own forms, or if the study results will be presented or published in any public venue, institutional review board (IRB) approval should be obtained prior to data harvesting.

Step 1: Identify an Outcome, and Form the Question (Chapter 7)

In this pilot study, the following PICO question can be used to examine the types and measurability of patient goals.

What are the distribution and measurability of impairment, functional limitation, and social goals in the initial visit documentation for patients with [insert a diagnosis of interest] in this [identify type of health-care facility] setting treated by this therapist?

P For patients with (a particular diagnosis), treated in this (specify type) facility, by this therapist

I who have impairment

C functional

C social goals

O What is the frequency of goals in each disablement category?

O What is the frequency of measurable goals in each category?

Remember to pick a diagnosis that is common to your practice or one that presents particular challenges. Licensed clinicians should review the records of patients who were managed personally, including the write-up of the initial evaluation. Nonlicensed clinicians, or those who do not have access to patient records, may use the data set provided in Appendix 3 to complete the exercise for a diagnostic group of personal interest.

Use the Model for Rehabilitation Services Delivery to organize this question as it relates to your practice setting. A sample is provided in Appendix 2.

Step 2: Conduct a Search of the Literature (Chapter 8)

The purpose of conducting a literature review is to determine if the question has been answered previously or to determine how others have tried to study the question. The literature may help to refine the question or clarify what data should be harvested.

Identify search terms for each component of the PICO/PIO question. Searching individual terms and then combining search results should provide a reasonable review of available literature. Remember to search multiple databases for journal articles, guidelines, systematic reviews, and diagnosis-specific websites. Print the history of each search in order to document the methods used to answer the question.

In this question, key words should probably include:

- *Diagnosis* (and any synonyms or abbreviations for that diagnosis)
- *Impairment*
- *Goals*
- *Functional goals*
- *Functional limitations*
- *Social/role goals*
- *Disability goals*
- *Practice setting* (*specify your own type*)
- *Outcomes*
- *Physical therapy*

If the question has been studied, you will need to determine how closely a published study parallels practice in your own setting. If no literature is found, then you should use the related literature to identify how others study individual aspects of the question and whether your practices parallel measurement or goal-setting trends in the literature.

Step 3: Identify a Rationale for Conducting the Study and Potential Action Plans (Chapter 8)

Write the rationale for conducting this study. It should address what outcomes will be investigated and how the answer to the study question will improve service delivery in your specific setting.

Avoid global statements such as, "This study will allow me to improve patient care by making me more aware of my goal writing." Increased awareness can result from reviewing two or three charts, without having to convert documentation into data. Provide at least three **reasons** why this study will be helpful for improving practice:

1.
2.
3.

It may be helpful to make **predictions** about what the outcomes will be:

- What percentage of the total goals will be impairment goals?   ___%
- What percentage of the total goals will be functional goals?   ___%
- What percentage of the impairment goals will be measurable? ___%
- What percentage of the functional goals will be measurable?   ___%

Describe how the results will translate into actions that can be taken in your practice setting. These **action plans** should be realistic for the setting, acknowledging the structure and processes of practice patterns and the personnel involved.

1. Describe what actions will be taken if the results *match* predictions.
2. Describe what actions will be taken if the results *exceed* predictions.
3. Describe what actions will be taken if the results are *lower* than the predictions or are inconclusive.

Step 4: Define Relevant Variable Codes (Chapter 9)

Based on the question components and the literature review, list the variables for which data will be collected. To the right, provide the operational definition of each level within each variable.

Name of Variable or Data Column	Code Levels	Operational Definition
e.g., Age	Number	Age of the child in months at the time of initial examination, or age of adult in years.
e.g., Sex	1	Female
	2	Male

A key with suggested codes is provided in Appendix 4.

Step 5: Create a Data Set (Chapter 10)

Use the PICO/PIO question and the coding handbook derived from the question and the literature to create a data collection form that includes all of the data to harvest. Use underlined fields where information will be recorded. Place codes directly on the form so the correct response can be circled. Both of these formats will allow you to scan the form for missing data and reduce translation errors when entering the data into a spreadsheet.

Review 10 or more charts of patients that fit the question. Complete one data collection form for each chart, and then transfer the data to a spreadsheet using the following format. Be sure to keep a list of subject ID numbers and the related chart in a separate, secure place.

Sample Data Collection Form

Coder's Name/Initials_____   Coding Date_____

Subject ID number _____

(Are number & patient name/chart number recorded on a separate, secure list? Y ___N___)

Pt. Age _____yrs

Clinic Site   1 = Site from which charts are accessed

                      2 = Identify any additional sites with a separate code

Sex: 1=F   1=M

Primary Diagnosis ICD 9 code   _____

Number of Impairment Goals   _____   Number measurable _____

Number of Functional Goals   _____   Number measurable _____

Number of Social Goals   _____   Number measurable _____

Total number of goals   _____   Number measurable _____

Exceptions and Notes:

The following is an example of a spreadsheet layout for this study. Note that there are no columns for totals because the spreadsheet can calculate them, but you can add totals if desired.

Subject ID	Age yrs	Clinic site	Sex	Dx	# Impairment goals	# Measurable impairment goals	# Function goals	# Measurable function goals	# Social goals	# Measurable social goals

Step 6: Analyze the Data (Chapter 11)

Using the data set (or the Sample Data Set in Appendix 3), answer the following to evaluate the quality of the data set:

1. Are there any missing data points? If so, describe a correction strategy.
2. Are there data points that appear incorrect? If so, review the data collection forms for transcription errors.

Refer to your PICO/PIO question as the starting point for data analysis. In the chart below, identify the variables, the statistical formulae needed to answer the question, the resulting type of answer, and any limitations to the data you can identify. One example for "age" is provided. Appendix 5 has this table worked out for the sample question.

Variable List	Statistic	Description of the Result	Actual Results	Limitations/ Notes
Age	Mean, standard deviation, and range	Average age and range of ages of sample in the study	Mean = 39.5 yrs SD = 16.79 Range = 16–69 yrs	May or may not be like those studied in the literature.

Perform a frequency count of the number of goals in each category (impairment, functional, and social). What can you say about the frequencies and distribution of the types and measurability of the goals?

Step 7: Interpret Results, and Create a Report (Chapter 12)

Use this checklist to create a final report of the outcome study.

Section of Report	Check-offs/Reminders
Introduction of the Problem	
PICO or PIO Question	
Rationale	
Search History Summary	
Literature Summary	
Was your question studied?	
Summarize literature on key variables.	
Methods	
Chart sampling process	
Sample description	
Statement of IRB approval (if appropriate)	
Definitions of variables and coding procedures	
Data Analysis Methods Summary	
Data Analysis Results Tables	
Sample	
Descriptive Summaries	
Correlations (if appropriate)	
Comparisons (if appropriate)	
Discussion	
Answer to the Question	
Integration of Literature with Study Results	
Strengths of the Study	
Limitations of the Study	
Recommendations for Service Delivery	

Model of Rehabilitation Services Delivery for Sample Question

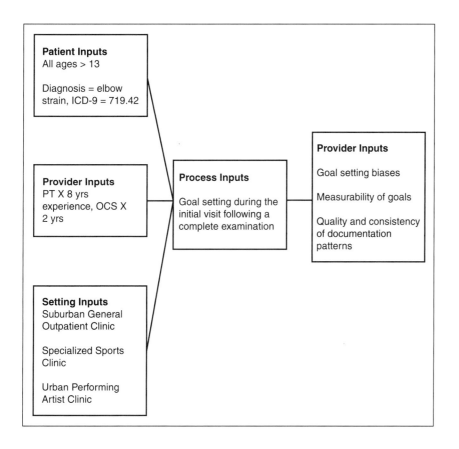

Patient Inputs
All ages > 13

Diagnosis = elbow
strain, ICD-9 = 719.42

Provider Inputs
PT X 8 yrs
experience, OCS X
2 yrs

Setting Inputs
Suburban General
Outpatient Clinic

Specialized Sports
Clinic

Urban Performing
Artist Clinic

Process Inputs

Goal setting during the
initial visit following a
complete examination

Provider Inputs

Goal setting biases

Measurability of goals

Quality and consistency
of documentation
patterns

Sample Data Set

Subject ID	Age (yrs)	Clinical Setting	Sex	Dx	# Impairment Goals	# Functional Goals	# Social Goals	Total Goals	# Measurable Impairment Goals	# Measurable Functional Goals	# Measurable Social Goals
01	18	1	1	719.42	2	2	1	5	2	1	0
02	40	2	2	719.42	2	4	1	7	2	1	1
03	47	3	1	719.42	5	1	1	7	4	0	1
04	37	3	2	719.42	3	2	2	7	3	2	1
05	22	1	1	719.42	1	2	1	4	1	1	0
06	53	2	1	719.42	4	2	2	8	2	1	0
07	45	3	2	719.42	4	3	0	7	4	2	0
08	69	2	1	719.42	0	4	0	4	0	1	0
09	48	1	1	719.42	2	4	1	7	1	1	1
10	16	3	2	719.42	3	1	2	6	1	2	1

Sample Codes and Operational Definitions

Name of Variable or Data Column	Code	Operational Definition
Subject ID	1–10	Sequential numbers as record is reviewed
Age	yrs	Age in years based on previous birthday
Clinical Setting	1	Suburban sports clinic
	2	Suburban general adult outpatient
	3	Urban performing artist clinic
Sex	1	Female
	2	Male
Diagnoses	111.11	ICD 9 code of primary diagnosis
# of Impairment Goals	#	A number count of goals that focus on impairment changes
# of Functional Goals	#	A number count of goals that focus on function changes
# of Social/Role Goals	#	A number count of goals that focus on social/role participation changes
Total # of Goals/Record	#	Total impairment, functional, and social goals
# of Measurable Impairment Goals	#	Total impairment goals that have a numerical goal, an objective method of measurement, or written with an "all-or-none" performance criterion
# of Measurable Functional Goals	#	Total functional goals that have a numerical goal, an objective method of measurement, or written with an "all-or-none" performance criterion
# of Measurable Social/ Role Goals	#	Total social/role goals that have a numerical goal, an objective method of measurement, or written with an "all-or-none" performance criterion

Sample Data Calculations

Variable List	Statistic	Description of the Result	Actual Results	Limitations/ Comments
Age	Mean, standard deviation, and range	Average age and range of ages of sample in the study	Mean =39.5 yrs SD = 16.79 Range = 16–69 yrs	May or may not be like those studied in the literature
Clinical Setting	Frequency count	Number of patients from each setting	Sports clinic = 3 General outpt = 3 Performing arts = 4	
Sex	Frequency count	Number of each in the sample	1 = 6 Females 2 = 4 Males	
Diagnoses	Frequency	Frequency distribution	10 = 719.42	
# Impairment Goals	Sum (% total goals)		26 (42%)	
# Functional Goals	Sum (% total goals)		25 (40%)	
# Social Goals	Sum (% total goals)		11 (18%)	
Total # Goals	Sum of all goals		62	
# Measurable Impairment Goals	Sum (percentage of total impairment goals)		20/26 = (77%)	
# Measurable Functional Goals	Sum (% total functional goals)		12/25 = (48%)	
# Measurable Social Goals	Sum (% total social goals)		5/12 = (42%)	All goals = return to work or school

A Sample Pilot Study

The following section presents portions of a pilot outcome study conducted by George Gabriel, PT, DPT, which helps to illustrate the steps of outcome measurement described in prior chapters. This selection is presented as one person's exploration into documentation patterns and is not meant to represent the only "right answers" that result from conducting an outcome study. Additionally, this study was conducted as a course project during a single academic semester, so the number of charts and the amount of literature reviewed are artificially limited by the constraints of time. When conducting a study in the clinical setting, the investigating clinician will need to consider a larger sample size and a more thorough review of the literature.

Clarifying comments and alternate approaches to selected parts of the study are presented in boxes. These comments may expand on what is presented in the text or serve as a reminder of points to consider. In all cases, if you need more explanation, refer to the respective chapter(s) in the text.

The sample illustrates the same question that is suggested as a starting point for clinicians who are just starting outcome research based on their own clinical data. Keep in mind that the results and conclusions of every study will be different based on the diagnosis of interest, the clinicians whose records are reviewed, the type and demands of the setting in which the clinicians are documenting, and the literature reviewed by the investigating clinician.

A SAMPLE STUDY OF DOCUMENTATION PATTERNS

George L. Gabriel, PT, DPT, with book adaptations and comments by Sandra L. Kaplan, PT, PhD

QUESTION

For patients with a diagnosis of low back pain managed by this physical therapist in an urban hospital, outpatient setting, who have impairment and functional goals established during the initial visit, what is the frequency and measurability of each category of goal?

In PICO/PIO Format

> P: For patients with a diagnosis of low back pain managed by this physical therapist in an urban hospital, outpatient setting,
>
> I: who have impairment and functional goals established during the initial visit,
>
> O: what is the frequency of each type of goal?
>
> O: what is the measurability of each type of goal?

> **Comment:** *In this case, the question is phrased as a PIO question, with the intent to describe the results without a comparison component. The question could also be phrased as follows if the clinician were interested in comparing the frequencies:*
> - *P: For patients with a diagnosis of low back pain managed by this physical therapist in an urban hospital, outpatient setting,*
> - *I: who have impairment goals,*
> - *C: and functional goals established during the initial visit,*
> - *O: what is the difference in frequencies of each type of goal?*
> - *O: what is the difference in measurability of each type of goal?*

RATIONALE

Third-party payers have pressured physical therapists to support the benefits of their services in producing functional change in order to be reimbursed. In an effort to track functional outcomes, the trend is to design functional and measurable goals at the initial exam stage and assess achievement at follow-up through discharge. Although the general consensus may lean toward the idea that this is normal practice, there may still be a tendency to treat and document change in patients based on impairments (Soukup & Vollestad, 2001).

> **Comment:** *Other reasons for conducting a study of patient goals have included the need to identify how function is currently measured, to identify standards for assessment that might not be currently used in the clinical setting, to validate current practice, and to streamline expectations of how goals are documented within a single setting. The rationale identifies the problem and reasons for trying to solve the problem, and these form the basis for potential action plans.*

ACTION PLAN

The goals of this study are to determine individual goal writing practices and compare them with those in the current literature in the hopes that consistency with current practice would be discovered. If this is not found, this study may serve as a catalyst for self-monitoring and for in-service training at the individual's setting.

> **Comment:** *A plan of action (self-monitoring and in-service training) addresses how the data will be used to improve practice. Other plans might address altering documentation formats to promote inclusion of functional goals generated by the patient, collecting additional data from the same clinician to see if trends in documentation persist, collecting additional data from other clinicians in the same setting to see if others are as variable as the investigating clinician. It is important to identify an action plan before moving ahead with an outcome study. The action plans clarify what the clinician can possibly do with the results to improve practice and help to frame the study's role for quality improvement processes.*

REVIEW OF LITERATURE

> **Comment:** *The review of literature is not presented in its entirety; it has been edited to present sample summaries that relate to the question. The content and organization of the review of literature will differ for each study according to the interests, setting and needs of the investigating clinician.*

Search Strategy

Two strategies were used to search the literature for this study: an electronic database search using OVID and VALE (to search Medline from 1996 to the present, CINAHL, all EBM reviews, HealthSTAR, and PsycINFO) and citation tracking. Keywords included: low back pain, mechanical low back pain, physical therapy, physiotherapy, outcomes, goals, and quality of life. To be accepted, an article had to be no more than 5 years old (1998-present), unless the topic of study closely pertained to the question.

Nine articles were read for this study, which included two systematic reviews (Guzman, et al., 2001; Karjalainen, et al., 2001), three outcome studies (Fisher & Hardie, 2002; Riddle, Stratford, & Binkley, 1998; Soukup & Vollestad, 2001), a case study (Deyo, et al., 2000), and three clinical trials (Moffet, et al., 1999; Sullivan, Shoaf, & Riddle, 2000; Weiner, et al., 2003).

Subjects Studied

The description of subjects varied, with the most common descriptor being the mean age and one study reporting the median age (Soukup & Vollestad, 2001). Mean ages were closely matched in five studies and ranged from the late 30s to early 40s (Fisher & Hardie, 2002; Karjalainen, et al., 2001; Moffet, et al., 1999; Riddle, et al., 1998; Sullivan, et al., 2000).

> **Comment:** *It is important to identify who have been studied to determine if they are similar to the subjects in one's own pilot data. In addition to age, it may be useful to know something about the duration of their diagnoses and the settings in which they were treated.*

Impairment vs. Functional Goals

The intervention being studied in the PICO question is goal-writing trends. All but one article (Riddle, et al., 1998) included impairment goals or measures concerning pain. Lumbar flexion (Sullivan, et al., 2000), postural control (Weiner, et al., 2003), mobility, strength, fitness (Guzman, et al., 2001; Karjalainen, et al., 2001), and back endurance (Guzman, et al.) were also measured.

In searching for functional goals, little was found in the form of actual goals. Only two articles cited vague functional goals, including transfers, stair negotiation, and ambulation (Fisher & Hardie, 2002), functional reach, lifting, and balance (Weiner, et al., 2003). The majority of the literature involved functional measurement tools. The Roland-Morris Back Pain Questionnaire was used in over 50% of the studies (Guzman, et al., 2001; Moffett, et al., 1999; Riddle, et al., 1998; Sullivan, et al., 2000; Weiner, et al.). The Oswestry

Low Back Pain Disability Questionnaire was used in two studies (Fisher & Hardie; Karjalainen, et al., 2001), and the Sickness Impact Profile was used in two studies (Guzman, et al.; Karjalainen, et al.).

METHODS/SUBJECTS

The records of 10 patients who had been diagnosed with low back pain and treated by this physical therapist in a hospital-based, outpatient physical therapy clinic are included in the data. The therapist used daily records and a documentation database of patients treated during the past year to find the 10 subjects. The inclusion criteria were that the original diagnosis had to be low back pain, and the patient had to have been initially examined by the researching therapist. No patient was excluded from the original 10 found.

> **Comment:** *Even though the clinician indicated who or which charts are eligible to be in the study (the P section of the PICO/PIO question), it is critical to identify who was actually included to identify any unexpected sampling biases.*

RESULTS

Table 1 presents the raw data for the 10 charts that were reviewed. Goals were categorized as impairment goals if the focus of change was at the tissue or body level and as functional goals if the focus of change was an activity or skill. Goals were categorized as measurable if the expected change was written with a numerical endpoint or if the activity was a criterion referenced "all or none" response. Goals written with up or down arrows, "will increase," or "will improve" were not considered measurable as a specific endpoint was not identified.

Table 1.

Raw Data							
Subject ID	Age (yrs)	Sex	Dx	# Impairment Goals	# Function Goals	# Measurable Impairment Goals	# Measurable Function Goals
Y01	57	1	724.2	2	1	2	1
Y02	42	1	724.2	1	2	1	2
Y03	32	2	724.2	2	3	2	3
Y04	31	2	724.2	2	2	2	1
Y05	31	1	724.2	3	0	2	0
Y06	33	1	724.2	2	1	2	1
Y07	32	1	724.2	2	2	2	2
Y08	55	1	724.2	3	1	3	1
Y09	45	2	724.2	3	2	3	2
Y10	45	1	724.2	2	2	2	2

Table 2 illustrates the mean age of this sample as 40.3 years, which falls into the range of the sample found in the literature. Thirty percent were male, and 70% were female. The mean duration of pain for 8 subjects in the sample was 2.98 years.

Table 2.

Description of Subjects' Age, Gender		
Data Set	Mean Age (yrs)	Gender (%)
N = 10	40.3	F: 70% M: 30%

A total of 22 impairment goals was written, with a mean of 2.2 goals per patient. A total of 16 functional goals was written, with a mean of 1.6 goals per patient. All goals were evaluated for measurability. Of the 22 impairment goals, 21 were deemed measurable (96%). Fifteen of the 16 functional goals were also measurable (94%). See Table 3 for details.

Table 3.

Distribution of Types and Measurability of Goals				
Descriptive Stats	Impairment Goals	Functional Goals	Measurable Impairment Goals	Measurable Functional Goals
Sum	22	16	21	15
Frequency	58%	42%	96%	94%

Comment: A narrative explanation of what is in the tables if very helpful to the reader, particularly if the report will be seen by outside parties.

DISCUSSION

The sample data collected from a random search of 10 patients indicate that for patients with a diagnosis of low back pain managed by the researching therapist in an urban hospital, outpatient, clinical setting, who have impairment and functional goals, 58% of all goals are impairment, 42% are functional, 96% of impairment goals are measurable, and 94% of functional goals are measurable.

An initial prediction was made estimating percentages of impairment (50%), functional (50%), and measurable goals (75%). A 50/50 prediction of impairment versus functional goals was probably a safe bet but turned out to be fairly close. The outstanding percentage of measurable goals written was a pleasant finding.

Primary Findings

1. I write more impairment goals and less functional goals than I thought.
2. I write more measurable goals than I thought.
3. I do not use any functional measurement tools of any kind for any of my outpatients. These tools would be helpful for legitimately tracking outcomes and may help facilitate functional goal writing for my patients.

> **Comment:** *It is helpful to summarize who was studied and what was found to answer the original PICO/PIO question. The following sections can then interpret the usefulness of the study, what was learned from the literature that might improve the outcomes of the study, and recommended action plans based on what was learned from the study. The above findings were written in the first person as the author was writing this paper for a class assignment. This informal approach might be fine for an internal report or for a report to colleagues in an educational forum. If the report were going to be viewed by outside parties, it would be more appropriate to summarize the findings without personal reference. For example:*
> *1. More impairment goals and less functional goals are written than were predicted.*
> *2. Goals were more measurable than predicted.*

The low percentage of functional goals is probably not coincidental. There are certainly some diagnoses for which the chronic nature makes it difficult to formulate functional goals. The quality of goal-writing is affected by many factors, including the day's caseload, administrative duties, and staffing, to name just a few.

The review of literature was conducted to find current evidence on the frequency and measurability of impairment and functional goal-writing. The one tool that was most often cited was the Roland-Morris Back Pain Questionnaire. Based on some preliminary evidence, this appears to be a valid and reliable tool specific to back pain diagnosis and may be used for tracking functional change in patients who suffer from low back pain.

Limitations

A limitation of this study may be the broadness of the diagnosis chosen in the original question. Specifying a characteristic of the duration (i.e., acute, sub-acute, chronic) of low back pain and/or a pain etiology (i.e., HNP, stenosis) may have better focused the search; however, the search yielded a narrow collection regardless. This may also be a result of the limited search strategy.

> **Comment:** *Always include the limitations of the methods, the data, and thus the application of the data as a basis for clinical decision-making. A key limitation to any pilot study is the small sample size, as that by itself may produce type I and II errors. On the other hand, even a small retrospective pilot study can yield valid evidence about practice patterns that can be used as the basis for improvement.*

RECOMMENDATIONS

1. Organize a team that includes both clinicians and management to further research the Roland-Morris Back Pain Questionnaire and other functional outcome tools best suited for this setting's patient population, and decide on the most appropriate. The staff may have to be trained in its use.

2. Consider expanding the data set to include patient records from other staff in the same clinical setting to see if the percentage distributions of goals and their measurability hold up.

3. Consider repeating this study on a different diagnostic group prevalent in this setting to identify the percentage distributions of goals and their measurability and to identify measurement trends in the literature.

4. Consider training other clinical staff in the processes for conducting these studies in order to facilitate greater buy-in for changes that are recommended as a result of these studies.

Comment: *These are sample recommendations that have come from a variety of clinicians. The individual clinician should make only recommendations that will realistically work in his/her own clinical setting; recommendations need to account for available resources, clinician and administration interests in improving services, administrative processes, and the costs of implementing recommendations.*

References

Deyo, R.A., Schall, M., Berwick, D.M., Nolan, T., & Carver, P. (2000). Continuous quality improvement for patients with back pain. Journal of General Internal Medicine. 15, 647–655.

Fisher, K., & Hardie, R.J. (2002). Goal attainment scaling in evaluating a multidisciplinary pain management programme. Clinical Rehabilitation,16, 871–877.

Guzman, J., Esmail, R., Karjalainen, K., Malmivaara, A., Irwin, E., & Bombardier, C. (2001). Multidisciplinary rehabilitation for chronic low back pain: systematic review. British Medical Journal, 322, 1511–1516.

Karjalainen, K., Malmivaara, A., van Tulder, M., Roine, R., Jauhiainen, M., Hurri, H. & Koes, B. (2001). Multidisciplinary biopsychosocial rehabilitation for subacute low back pain in working-age adults: a systematic review within the framework of the Cochrane Collaboration Back Review Group. Spine, 26, 262–269.

Moffet, J.K., Torgerson, D., Bell-Syer, S., Jackson, D., Llewlyn-Philips, H., Farrin, A., & Barber J.

(1999). Randomized controlled trial of exercise for low back pain: clinical outcomes, costs, and preferences. British Medical Journal, 319, 279–283.

Riddle, D.L., Stratford, P.W., & Binkley, J.M. (1998). Sensitivity to change of the Roland-Morris Back Pain Questionnaire: Part 2. Physical Therapy, 78, 1197–1207.

Soukup, M.G., & Vollestad, N.K. (2001). Classification of problems, clinical findings and treatment goals in patients with low back pain using the ICIDH-2 beta-2. Disability and Rehabilitation, 23, 463–472.

Sullivan, M.S., Shoaf, L.D., & Riddle, D.L. (2000). The relationship of lumbar flexion to disability in patients with low back pain. Physical Therapy, 80, 240–250.

Weiner, D.K., Rudy, T.E., Glick, R.M., Boston, J. R., Lieber, S.J., Morrow, L.A., & Taylor S. (2003). Efficacy of percutaneous electrical nerve stimulation for the treatment of chronic low back pain in older adults. Journal of the American Geriatric Society, 51, 599–608.

Answer Key to Exercises (Chapters 5, 6, and 7)

Chapter 5 Exercise Key

Item	Classification	Factors Increasing Limitation	Factors Decreasing Limitation
Inability to button shirts	Functional limitation	Smaller buttons or buttonholes; less time to complete the task	Larger buttons or buttonholes; substitute Velcro for buttons; more time to complete the task
Inability to put on shoes	Functional limitation	Thick socks; laces on shoes; less time to complete task	Thinner socks; slip-on or Velcro shoes; use of shoehorn; more time to complete task
Wrist edema/ swelling	Impairment	Repetitive injury conditions; restrictive clothing/jewelry	Wraps; hand position; use of thermal agents
Frequent spillage when attempting to cook	Functional limitation	Heavy utensils/pots; upper extremity weakness; visual impairments; height of work surface; inadequate balance	Lighter or smaller utensils/pots; upper extremity strength; visual accommodation; decrease height of work surface; sit while preparing food
Inability to attend church	Participation restriction	Deconditioning; lack of transportation; poor building access; fear of falling	Improved strength and endurance; transportation; alternate access to building; improved balance and use of adaptive equipment
Weak grasp	Impairment	Weight of objects to lift/manipulate; less time to perform task or number of repetitions required in task	Strengthen hand; reduce weight of items to be lifted; break tasks into smaller parts; use adaptive equipment to assist

Chapter 6 Exercise Key

Example 1:

<u>Inputs:</u> Children with cerebral palsy

<u>Processes:</u> Functional physical therapy and therapy were based on the principle of normalization of the quality of movement

<u>Outputs:</u> Motor abilities

Example 2:

<u>Inputs:</u> Two groups of patients who had hemiplegia secondary to stroke

<u>Processes:</u> Balance and mobility retraining by physical therapy with and without the addition of NeuroCom Balance Master

<u>Outputs:</u> Berg Balance Scale and the Timed Up & Go test measures

Example 3:

<u>Inputs:</u> Individuals with COPD

<u>Processes:</u> Pulmonary rehabilitation program

<u>Outputs:</u> Changes in QOL

Chapter 7 Exercise Key

Question 1. What are the levels of patient satisfaction following 2 and 4 weeks of intervention by patients with acute plantar fasciitis? Depending on who is asking the question, this can be an outcome measure for either the individual provider who wants feedback from patients or the management of a setting who wants to know about the satisfaction levels of all patients in that sample group, regardless of clinician assignment.

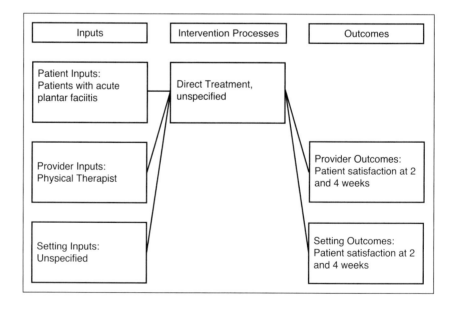

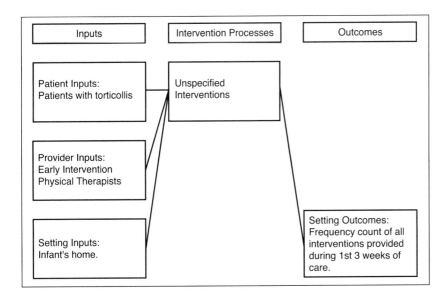

Question 2. What interventions are utilized by early intervention therapists for infants with torticollis during the first 3 weeks of home visits? A frequency count will provide a broad description of what services are provided. As more than one therapist is included in the sample, this represents an administrative or setting outcome.

Question 3. The P is very broad, the I and C reflect different intervention activities but are not very specific, and the O has 2 outcomes, neither of which is measurable. An improved version of the question might look like this:

P: For young children (ages 3–5 years) with cerebral palsy who receive physical therapy services at home

I: does sustained stretching of the knee flexors

C: or progressive resistance strengthening of the knee extensors

O: improve stride length during gait?

Question 4. The P is a bit broad. The I and C are reasonably defined, but the O is not measurable. The concept of "easier overhead reaching" will need to be defined operationally for height or shoulder flexion range. Additionally, the change in score does not result in a change in function; rather, a change in pain level from interventions and healing results in functional changes. Thus, looking for a correlation rather than a cause and effect/result would be the better orientation. An improved version might look like this:

P: For adults with chronic rotator cuff injuries of longer than 6 months, managed in an outpatient facility

I: does a change of 2 points on a visual analogue scale

C: compared with a 4-point change

O: correlate with achievement of 150° of overhead reaching?

Question 5. The patient description is too broad; the outcome is not a measurement, rather, a descriptor that belongs with the intervention. Pain level is the measured outcome, but when the measure is taken needs to be identified. The question could be better organized as follows:

P: For my patients (with some specific diagnosis or characteristics)

I: who receive ultrasound for 2 weeks of treatment

O: how does the pain level change (at what time of measurement)?

Glossary

Access satisfaction—Perceptions of the convenience with which services are scheduled, the hours of service, the distance to service, and perceived availability (Rees Lewis, 1994).

Atmospherics—Perceptions of the environment in which services are delivered.

Benchmarking—Process of comparing one's own procedures and outcomes with a known or best available gold standard in order to improve consumer or client service outcomes.

Care paths—Documentation mechanisms that indicate if the clinical pathway has been followed.

Clinical pathways—Sometimes called critical pathways, outline of agreed-upon steps for the diagnosis and interdisciplinary management of a condition or procedure for individual patients.

Clinical significance—Changes in a measured variable that result in useful changes.

Cohort data—Measurements taken from a group of patients with similar characteristics.

Comparative statistics—Determine whether two or more groups of data are different and suggest cause-and-effect relationships between an intervention and an outcome.

Continuous quality improvement (CQI)—Ongoing process of measuring the quality of services provided and making the services more effective (Coleman & Endsley, 1999; McIntosh, May, & Stymiest, 1994).

Correlative statistics—Describe relationship of changes in one variable to changes in another variable.

Cost-benefit—Positive benefits of providing services relative to the cost or negative aspects of providing the service (Thompson & Cohen, 1990).

Cost-effectiveness—Comparison of the cost to produce the same outcome by similar providers or service delivery systems.

Cost-utility—Estimates of patient preferences for different health states relative to the length and quality of life and available interventions (Haas, 1993; Luce & Simpson, 1995).

Criterion reference—Observations or measurements that reflect the patient's performance of an activity as compared with a task analysis of that activity.

Data harvesting—Process of identifying the measures of interest in records to create a data set.

Data mining—Process of exploring large data sets.

Data recording form—Form to record data on the variables of interest; useful for reducing data omissions and translation errors.

Data set—Collection of organized observations and measurements.

Descriptive statistics—Distribution of data points for a variable or category.

Dissemination—Process of presenting ideas or study results publicly.

Documentation—Process or products of recording the status, clinical decision-making, and the provision of health services.

Episode of intervention—Services provided without interruption for a patient condition or problem, generally marked by an initial evaluation at the start and a discharge summary at the end.

Evaluate-and-treat approach—Approach to patient care that is oriented toward the identification of impairments and/or deviations from normal function and the linking of these deviations to interventions that can address them.

Experimental bias—Imbalance of data that occurs when either the participants or the investigators have expectations for outcomes because either party knows who or what is being studied.

Fix-it approach—A stereotype of practice in which the focus of care is on curing, alleviating, or modifying patient problems and using normal health as the standard of comparison (Lynn & DeGrazia, 1991).

Functional limitation—Loss of the ability to perform tasks or activities.

Functional outcome—Measure of the patient's ability to perform the tasks of everyday living following an episode of intervention.

Goods satisfaction—Satisfaction with a product or item that can be used regardless of where it is produced.

Health-care outcomes—Results of patient or health service delivery.

Health-related quality of life—Multidimensional assessment of life satisfaction as it relates to the person's state of health and the societal expectations of people who do or do not have disabilities (Jenkins, 1992; Hoffman, Rouse, & Brin, 1995).

Historical bias—Imbalance in the data resulting from an event that happens outside of the patient care interaction and that might influence some aspect of patient care service or the measured outcomes.

Humaneness satisfaction—Patient's perception of the provider's warmth, caring, willingness to listen, appropriateness of nonverbal and verbal behaviors, and respect for the patient (Rees Lewis, 1994).

Impairment—Loss or abnormality at the tissue or organ level resulting in such changes as limited range of motion, decreases in strength or endurance, and postural malalignment.

Impairment outcomes—Measures of changes at the body or tissue level that may occur as a result of intervention.

Intervention—Any process or activity that occurs to or on behalf of a patient; may include direct or hands-on treatment, patient education, adaptation of the environment or of equipment.

Measurement bias—Imbalance in the data resulting from the choice of a measurement tool, from inherent errors associated with the application or recording of the measure, from limits of tool construction (e.g., selection of the items in a tool that create ceiling or floor affects), and from variations in documentation on the measure.

Medical effectiveness—Extent to which a medical intervention is able to cure a disease or condition.

Model of Rehabilitation Services Delivery—Graphic representation of the inputs, processes, and outcomes representative of physical therapy practice.

Model—Graphic or physical representation of a theory.

Morbidity—Ratio of sick to well in a community or to the frequency of complications that follows a medical intervention.

Mortality—Rate of death.

Normative standard—Observations or measurements that reflect the normal distribution of a characteristic in the general population.

Outcomes—Meaningful results following an episode of intervention.

Outcome approach—Approach to patient care in which meaningful goals are identified and resources and interventions are selected to manage the patient toward those goals.

Outcome measures—Wide variety of objective processes or tools used to measure patient status over time.

Outcome project manager—Person who organizes the activities of an outcomes study.

Outcome research—the systematic measurement of patient or service results.

Participation—Ability to fulfill personal and societal roles.

Patient outcomes—Changes in the consequences of illness or injury that occur as a result of intervention and that are meaningful to the patient.

Patient satisfaction—Patient's perceptions of the care he/she has received.

PICO—Acronym in evidence-based practice approaches to organize the components of an answerable, comparative question; Patient, Interventions, Comparison interventions, Outcomes.

PIO—Acronym in evidence-based practice approaches to organize the components of an answerable, descriptive question; Patient, Interventions, Outcomes.

Practice guidelines—Recommendations for patient management that are not unique to any one institution; that are established to improve patient outcomes, reduce wrongful management of patient conditions, control costs, and inform patients and clinicians about appropriate choices for medical management (Scalzitti, 2001; Woolf, 1992).

Procedure variability—Range of methods used by clinicians to perform the same task or to achieve the same endpoint.

Project costs—Direct and indirect expenses, including time, required to conduct an outcome study.

Protocols—Progression of a specific intervention for a particular diagnostic group initiated by a service provider within a specific discipline.

Provider outcomes—Results of service delivery activities, whether the provider is an individual or a group, that are meaningful to the providing clinician(s).

QALY—Assessment of duration of life weighed against the quality of that life.

Q-TWiST—Quality-adjusted Time Without Symptoms and Toxicities; a quality-adjusted survival analysis.

Quality assurance—Process used to monitor whether predetermined standards of service delivery are actually met in daily practice that has traditionally emphasized the correction of errors or the identification of poor performers.

Quality of life—A person's assessment of satisfaction with life.

Reflective practitioner—Someone who continually evaluates his or her effectiveness as a physical therapist (Tichenor & Davidson, 1997).

Relational database—Software design for managing complex collections of data.

Relative standard—Observations or measurements that reflect changes based on initial measurements and where the starting or ending points may be different for each person.

Retrospective chart review—Process of harvesting selected data from patient charts or files after patient has discontinued services.

Sampling bias—Imbalance of one or more characteristics in a group of patients studied.

Service outcomes—Results of the delivery of services within an institution, among similar institutions, or across larger health-care systems.

Service satisfaction—A patient's perceptions of satisfaction derived from interacting with a service provider.

Social/role limitations—Loss of ability to fulfill personal and societal roles.

Spreadsheet—Paper or software design for managing rows of data organized under labeled variable columns.

Statistical significance—Results of data analysis that exceed the level of chance.

Technical satisfaction—Patient's perceptions that the provider is knowledgeable and able to perform the necessary examination, evaluation, and treatment procedures in a comfortable and efficient way (Goldstein, et al., 2000).

Theory—Description of the relationships among concepts, structures, or phenomena.

Therapeutic indicators—Observations of patient characteristics; used by clinicians to determine the impact of interventions.

Total quality management (TQM)—Participatory and systematic approach to planning and implementing continuous organizational improvement focused on customer satisfaction (Kaluzny, et al., 1992).

Transformed data—Raw data that are converted to a different format for analysis or reporting, such as conversion of actual age to age groups.

Unit cost—Cost to produce or deliver one unit of a product or service; incorporates both direct and indirect costs of production.

Index

SCHOOL OF PHYSICAL THERAPY
TEXAS WOMAN'S UNIVERSITY
6700 FANNIN STREET
HOUSTON, TEXAS 77030-2343
TEL (713)794-2070
FAX (713)794-2071